# Take Control
# of Your
# IBS

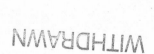

# Take Control of Your IBS

# IBS

## THE COMPLETE GUIDE TO MANAGING YOUR SYMPTOMS

Professor Peter Whorwell

**Vermilion**
LONDON

1 3 5 7 9 10 8 6 4 2

Vermilion, an imprint of Ebury Publishing,
20 Vauxhall Bridge Road,
London SW1V 2SA

Vermilion is part of the Penguin Random House group of companies
whose addresses can be found at global.penguinrandomhouse.com

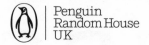

Penguin
Random House
UK

First published in the United Kingdom by Vermilion in 2017

www.penguin.co.uk

A CIP catalogue record for this book is available from the British Library

ISBN 9781785040405

616·362

Printed and bound in Great Britain by Clays Ltd, St Ives PLC

Penguin Random House is committed to a sustainable future for our
business, our readers and our planet. This book is made from Forest
Stewardship Council® certified paper.

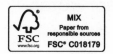

MIX
Paper from
responsible sources
FSC® C018179

Professor Whorwell has acted as a consultant for, or reviewed research grant
support from, the makers of some of the products mentioned in this book.

# CONTENTS

*I would like to thank all the doctors and researchers, too numerous to mention individually, who have worked in my team over the years and enabled me to build up a unit with an international reputation. Special thanks to my wife, Helen Carruthers, for illustrating the book so nicely and putting up with me during the process of writing it.*

# PREFACE

I have been a consultant gastroenterologist for over 30 years and have always enjoyed the challenge of trying to help people suffering from irritable bowel syndrome (IBS) and related conditions. There is no 'one-size-fits-all' treatment for IBS and, therefore, to effectively manage sufferers, the doctor has to spend a lot of time with each patient in order to work out which is the best treatment for that particular individual. Unfortunately, modern medicine has become a bit of a conveyer belt where a patient tends to be sidelined if they can't be fixed quickly and they continue to have symptoms, especially if all the tests are normal and the symptoms cannot be instantly explained, which is typical in IBS.

In addition, it must be virtually impossible for a patient to convey the complexity of their problem in a ten-minute consultation with their general practitioner. I often have to spend up to an hour with someone to establish exactly what is going on, so it must be very frustrating for both the patient and their general practitioner when they only have ten minutes in which to try and make some progress. Even if a patient is referred to a gastroenterologist, there are very few who specialise in the condition, which is a problem, as IBS is the most common gastrointestinal disorder they will encounter.

There are many misconceptions about IBS and this is partly because generations of medical students, including myself, have been taught that it is a psychological condition, mainly of rather delicate females, which can't be cured and the best treatment is lots of bran. Early on in my career,

I became very suspicious that bran actually made many IBS sufferers worse and subsequently published a study which showed that only 10 per cent of patients improved on bran, whereas 55 per cent got worse. I used to regularly see people who were advised to take bran and, when they told their doctor they thought it was making them worse, were told that this was because they weren't taking enough of the stuff. At that time, the idea that bran is good for you was so entrenched in society that, when a newspaper reported my views on bran, I got letters from the public saying I should be struck off the medical register for holding such an outrageous opinion.

Fortunately, more than 20 years after publishing that paper, the message finally seems to be sinking in. Hopefully, with the advent of the internet, such messages will get through more quickly in the future, although the one that IBS is not 'all psychological' seems to be taking its time. It still never ceases to amaze me how many patients tell me that they have been told that IBS is all in their head, sometimes on so many occasions that they even start to believe this total misrepresentation of the condition. Stress can make any medical condition worse and IBS is no exception, but it is not the cause.

It has to be acknowledged that IBS cannot be cured, but there is much that can be done to bring it under control by finding a combination of options that suit a particular individual. I will give anything a try, as long as it is safe. That is why I experimented with hypnotherapy, which to my surprise, turned out to be remarkably effective in reducing symptoms in up to 70 per cent of IBS patients. However, it has taken me a long time to convince my colleagues, many of whom initially greeted this treatment for IBS with considerable scepticism.

My Unit cares for approximately 3,000 patients with IBS every year and we also have a wide-ranging research programme investigating possible causes of the condition as well as how it affects people. In addition, we undertake trials of new treatment options such as dietary manipulation, behavioural techniques such as hypnotherapy and new medications. All this research has resulted in over 350 publications in a variety of prestigious journals and books.

I also act as a consultant to a number of pharmaceutical companies, strongly encouraging them to work in this field, which is so desperately in need of investment. In addition, I am an advisor for the UK's National Institute for Health and Care Excellence (NICE) where I help with the development of guidelines on the management of IBS. Consequently, I have huge experience of how to manage IBS, as well as of all the politics surrounding the subject, and the purpose of this book is to share that knowledge with you, in the hope that it will help you to manage your condition more effectively in the future.

# INTRODUCTION

Irritable bowel syndrome is an extremely common condition affecting as many as one in eight of the population, with women being affected more than men. The condition is found throughout the world and can affect any cultural or ethnic group. Luckily, the majority of sufferers only experience relatively mild symptoms and may not even have to visit their doctor. However, in a proportion of these people, their IBS is much more severe, with the condition profoundly affecting every aspect of their lives to the point where some can even become suicidal.

Unfortunately, the general public and even the medical profession often regard IBS as a purely psychological problem and certainly as nothing serious or anything to get worried about. Needless to say, nothing could be further from the truth but these misconceptions result in people making comments to sufferers such as, 'I have got IBS and I never have to see a doctor' or doctors telling them 'to pull themselves together' or 'It is all in the head.' Another problem is that the symptoms of IBS can vary enormously between different people, leading sufferers to say, 'My symptoms don't seem to match those of other people I know with IBS' or 'I have never met anybody with symptoms like mine.' Regrettably, once a diagnosis of IBS has been made, sufferers are often left on their own – 'You will just have to cope with it' – and are not taken seriously.

This book is designed to offer help to those people in this situation where, actually, there is much that can be done to bring the condition under control. Alternatively, you may have a partner or friend who is struggling with their IBS and you want to try and help them. Before trying to help yourself or others with the aid of this book, it is important that the diagnosis of IBS has been confirmed, as other conditions may have to be ruled out before embarking on a treatment programme.

As someone who still personally sees approximately 2,000 people affected by severe IBS every year, I remain convinced that education is an absolutely essential starting point in trying to manage this condition. If a sufferer fully understands the complexities of IBS, they can then 'pick and mix' from various treatment options available, as every person with IBS is different and responds differently to a particular treatment: one size certainly does not fit all.

Consequently, the first three chapters of this book are largely educational and possibly read a little like a textbook. The subsequent chapters are about diagnosis and treatment. It is difficult to direct all the information in the book to all IBS sufferers and some of the information will not necessarily be relevant to you in particular. Of course, you may feel that you know enough about the background to IBS, in which case feel free to start at Chapter 4. In order to ensure that each chapter can be read on its own, there is some repetition between chapters and I hope that this is not too distracting, but instead serves to consolidate your knowledge of this challenging disorder as you go through the book.

Irritable bowel syndrome cannot be cured, but over the years I have found that the vast majority of sufferers can learn to manage the condition to the extent that it becomes just a nuisance rather than a constant intrusion. I do hope this book helps you to take control of this condition which, if given a chance, can so easily take over your life.

# CHAPTER 1
# THE NORMAL GUT

## How the gut functions

Compared to the heart, which is just a glorified pump, the gastrointestinal system is extremely complicated, as we will see by what follows. When we chew our food, it is lubricated by saliva which contains enzymes – chemicals that break down food or bacteria – and it is then propelled down the oesophagus (also called the gullet) into the stomach where it is mixed with acid (gastric acid) and more enzymes (see Table 1 overleaf).

The acid helps to 'sterilise' the food and the enzymes start the process of digestion. The food in the stomach then has to be broken down into small pieces by the stomach before being delivered to the small intestine (or small bowel) where it is digested by different enzymes from the pancreas and the lining of the small intestine (see Table 1). In addition, bile, which is made in the liver, passes down the bile duct, into the small intestine where it helps to dissolve fats in a similar way to detergents. As the contents of the small intestine move further down, all the nutrients are absorbed into the bloodstream to be processed further and stored in the body. By the time the contents reach the large intestine (also called the large bowel or colon), most of the nutrients have been removed, leaving undigested material, such as fibre. It is the function of the colon to dry out these waste products and store them until they are ready to be passed into the toilet (opening one's bowels or defaecation).

---

**Table 1** Principal enzymes found in various parts of the gastrointestinal system and what type of food product they break down

| | |
|---|---|
| Saliva* | Amylase – starch |
| Stomach | Pepsin – protein |
| Pancreas | Trypsin – protein |
| | Chymotrypsin – protein |
| | Carboxypeptidase – protein |
| | Elastase – protein |
| | Amylase – starch |
| | Lipase – fat |
| Small intestine | Lactase – lactose |
| | Sucrase – sucrose |
| | Maltase – maltose |

\* Saliva also contains an enzyme called lysozyme that kills bacteria

---

## The mouth, pharynx and oesophagus

At the back of the mouth and nose there is a short tube called the pharynx which connects with the larynx (or voice box) and trachea (also called the windpipe) as well as with the oesophagus. A flap-like structure at the end of the pharynx called the epiglottis covers the larynx when we

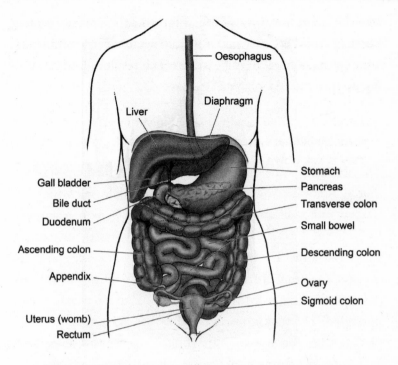

**Figure 1** The main parts of the gastrointestinal system and where they are in the body

swallow so that food goes down the oesophagus and cannot get into the lungs. When we breathe, the epiglottis opens up the larynx to allow air to reach the lungs.

The oesophagus is a tube that runs down through the chest and connects with the stomach after it has passed through the diaphragm. The diaphragm is a large sheet of muscle that separates the chest from the abdomen (or abdominal cavity) and is used for breathing. The diaphragm has a hole in it to allow the oesophagus to reach the stomach which lies directly below the diaphragm. This hole is called the diaphragmatic hiatus and, if a part of the stomach slides through this hole up into the chest, this is called a hiatus or diaphragmatic hernia. Hiatus hernias are very common and seldom cause problems although they can lead to heartburn as a result of acid refluxing up into the oesophagus (see page 53).

## The stomach

The stomach is the only part of the gastrointestinal system that is not tube shaped. It is an expandable sac which is shaped rather like a large comma and acts as a reservoir for our food which can then be slowly passed on to the small intestine. The stomach makes enzymes (see Table 1 on page 6) and hydrochloric acid, which is strong enough to damage the lining of the gastrointestinal system if it is not protected. The acid activates the enzymes to start the process of digestion and is very important in preventing infection by killing the germs in anything we swallow. The stomach lining makes mucus which covers all the cells and prevents the acid damaging them. If the production of mucus fails or is impaired by medications, particularly anti-inflammatory drugs, then a gastric ulcer can develop. The oesophagus is not so well protected from acid and, therefore, if acid refluxes up into the oesophagus it can lead to heartburn or even damage the lining, causing inflammation or sometimes ulceration. The small intestine protects itself by making bicarbonate which neutralises the acid as it comes out of the stomach. If this system doesn't work properly or the stomach makes too much acid, a duodenal ulcer can occur. Following a meal, the stomach has usually finished emptying within approximately three hours, although this may take longer after a very large meal or after a very fatty meal. Fat delays gastric (stomach) emptying and that is why we feel full for longer after fatty foods.

## The small intestine

The small intestine starts at the pylorus which is the outlet from the stomach. The small intestine is divided into three sections, starting with the duodenum which is approximately 30 centimetres (1 foot) long, followed by the jejunum and ileum which are 2.4 metres (8 feet) and 3 metres (10 feet) long respectively. Bicarbonate, pancreatic enzymes and bile enter the duodenum via the bile and pancreatic ducts and this is where the main part of digestion starts. The lining of the jejunum also makes some enzymes (see Table 1 on page 6) to help with digestion. The principal nutrients in the diet are proteins, carbohydrates and fats which cannot be absorbed through the gut unless they are broken down (digested) into their basic constituents. Consequently, proteins are reduced to amino acids, carbohydrates to monosaccharides and fats to fatty acids, and these products are then absorbed, mainly through the lining of the jejunum and, to a lesser extent, the ileum. Protein and carbohydrate have a calorific value of 4 calories per gram whereas fat generates 9 calories per gram, so it is easy to see why people gain more weight when they are on a fatty diet. The small bowel joins up with the colon on the right-hand side of the abdomen and the last few centimetres are called the terminal ileum. The terminal ileum is the only part of the bowel that absorbs vitamin B12 and bile. This is important because, if it doesn't work properly or is diseased, people can develop anaemia, due to B12 deficiency, or diarrhoea because, if bile reaches the colon, it acts like a laxative. After food has left the stomach, it takes approximately four hours to reach the colon. During this time, all the nutrients and other dietary constituents that we need, such as vitamins and iron, are extracted. However, other products that cannot be digested in the small bowel, such as some forms of dietary fibre, pass on into the colon.

## The colon

The first part of the colon is called the caecum and the last part is the rectum, which ends at the anus. The sections between the caecum and rectum are called the ascending, transverse, descending and sigmoid colon. The appendix is a small blind-ending tube about 7.5–10 centimetres (3–4 inches) long which opens into the caecum. When the small bowel contents reach the caecum they are usually still liquid, but as they pass round the colon water is extracted leading to the formation of solid material, which is then passed out through the anus as a formed motion (stool). The colon is approximately 1.2–1.5 metres (4–5 feet) long and it takes approximately 40 hours for the contents to pass through. The anus has muscle around it to stop faeces leaking out but when a person wants to open their bowels, the anus relaxes to allow the stools to be passed out (defaecation). The colon contains huge amounts of bacteria which account for 50 per cent of stool weight with the remainder being largely undigested products and cells from the small bowel. These products can be 'digested' (fermented) by the bacteria in the colon and actually provide 10–20 per cent of our calories. It is thought that this process might be more active in some people and this may explain why they may have more trouble losing weight than others.

## Control of gastrointestinal function

The activity of the whole length of the gastrointestinal system has to be very tightly co-ordinated so that the various parts of the system can switch on and off their particular function at the appropriate time. This is achieved by the combined action of muscles, nerves and hormones with the brain fine-tuning these responses.

### The muscles of the gut

To move its contents from mouth to anus, the gut has muscle around it which contracts in an orderly manner to propel the food along (this process is called peristalsis). The muscle in the gut and other hollow organs, such as the bladder and uterus, is called smooth muscle (or non-striated or involuntary muscle) and contracts without conscious control. In contrast, skeletal muscle (or striated or voluntary muscle) is the type of muscle that moves, for instance, our arms or legs and is under our control. The heart has another type of involuntary muscle (cardiac muscle) which is only found in the heart and differs from both smooth or skeletal muscle.

The muscular activity of the gut is often referred to as motility and, when it goes wrong, it is called dysmotility or a motility disorder. In the gullet the food goes down very quickly into the stomach and is prevented from coming back up (reflux) by a valve (or sphincter) which is a strip of muscle around the bottom of the oesophagus that can relax when it is necessary for food to go through. When this sphincter does not work properly acid can reflux into the gullet causing heartburn, which is a burning feeling behind the breast bone (sternum). The diaphragmatic hiatus also 'pinches' the oesophagus to some extent to help reduce reflux. Consequently, if the hiatus is bigger than it should be or there is a hiatus hernia, this can also lead to heartburn. The muscles in the stomach make it work rather like a cement mixer until the food is broken up and liquid enough to go through into the small intestine. The muscles in the small intestine work differently to allow the food to pass through more slowly to give the food time to be digested enough to be absorbed. The colonic muscles then put the brakes on so that the contents of the colon can gradually be dried out and become more and more solid until they come to a halt near the rectum. The anus is a sphincter at the end of the rectum which helps the faeces stay in place until the bowels need to be opened, when it relaxes.

## The nerves of the gut

Nerves can be considered as the wiring of the body and are divided into two different types: There are afferent nerves which send information from the body to the brain and efferent nerves which send instructions from the brain to the body. The gut contains a complicated network of these different types of nerves (the enteric nervous system) which control the activity of the muscles and also allow it to sense what is going on, so that it can respond appropriately. In some parts of the gut, especially at the top and bottom end, this sensory system lets us know what is going on, whereas in other parts we don't feel anything unless something has gone wrong. Consequently, we feel it when acid gets into our oesophagus (commonly called heartburn) or when the rectum is full and we need to go to the toilet. However, we don't generally feel anything as the food goes through the rest of the system, although we can sometimes hear it in the form of gurgling or bowel sounds (this is called borborygmi – for more on this, see page 36).

Another part of the sensory system in the lining of the gut allows it to know which chemicals and foods are present so it can change the amount of acid, enzymes and bile we are making according to what is needed, without us having any knowledge of what is going on. The enteric nervous system (referred to as the 'gut brain') can operate on its own, but also communicates with the brain, which monitors its activity and allows us to respond to what is happening in our gut, if necessary. Consequently, we can feel hunger, can tell when we have eaten enough or know when our bowels need emptying. When we think about eating, tasting or chewing food the brain activates the gut to get it ready to receive the meal. This is called the cephalic phase of digestion which we do not feel in any way except perhaps for an increase in saliva. However, as we will see later, this can be a problem in IBS as the gut is already overactive and, therefore, this cephalic stimulation can cause symptoms without any food being swallowed.

The autonomic nervous system is the network of nerves that control the gut as well as other day-to-day functions of the body, such as breathing, heart rate, temperature and blood pressure. This system normally works without us knowing anything about what it is doing, but it can become overactive in IBS and this explains why some people with IBS can sweat more than usual or experience palpitations as well as low blood pressure.

## Gut hormones

Hormones are chemicals that produce an effect on various parts of the body without the need for a nerve and, in general, reach their target via the bloodstream. Consequently, they take a little longer to produce an effect than a nerve which produces an almost instantaneous effect. There are several hormones that control gastrointestinal function such as secretin, cholecystokinin and gastrin. Gastrin is probably the most well known and is released when food enters the stomach and it then stimulates the lining of the stomach to make acid.

# What is a normal bowel habit?

The ideal bowel habit is once a day, first thing in the morning, but it is surprising how many people do not necessarily experience this pattern. Consequently, 'normal' is usually defined as somewhere between three times a day and three times a week. However, if someone is outside this range and it is not causing any trouble, then nothing necessarily has to be done about it.

One important trigger to opening the bowels is the so-called 'gastrocolonic response'. This is the sensation of the need to empty the bowel caused by food or liquids such as tea or coffee entering the stomach. This reflex is most active in the morning and then usually disappears for the rest of the day and explains why most of us need to empty our bowels after breakfast but not after other meals. As we will see later, this reflex is also abnormal in IBS (see page 29).

In addition to the frequency of the bowel habit, it is important to know about the appearance of what comes out (the faeces or stools). An ideal stool should look like a sausage but again there is great variation, so if sometimes they are a bit hard and like rabbit droppings or somewhat porridge-like, that can just be a reflection of what we have eaten recently. However, if they are regularly very hard and difficult to pass or very loose, this might indicate a problem. Colour can also vary from day to day and can change from dark brown to pale brown and this can also be affected by what has been eaten. Iron tablets can make the stools black, therefore, it is not surprising that foods that contain a lot of iron, such as spinach, can darken the stools. Occasionally, food such as sweetcorn or peas can appear in the stools apparently unaltered and this is not a cause for concern. Some red foods such as tomato skins can occasionally be mistaken for blood. Actual blood in the stools is most often associated with piles (haemorrhoids), a cut in the anus (a fissure) or a sore anus (for instance, after a bout of diarrhoea). However, blood in the stools should never be ignored until more sinister causes have been excluded. Bleeding from the top end of the gut (for example, from a stomach ulcer) makes the stools jet black rather than red and, again, should never be ignored. The lining of the colon makes mucus which is protective but also acts as a lubricant. Some people make more mucus than others and may sometimes pass jelly-like mucus with their stool or occasionally on its own. This is not a problem as long as it is not bloodstained, which could indicate some inflammation.

# Wind

It is completely normal for the gut to accumulate gas. We all swallow some air when we are eating or even when we are just swallowing saliva. Something as simple as using chewing gum can lead to excessive gas because it leads to more swallowing and, therefore, more air is swallowed. In addition, if the gum is sugar free, then the artificial sweeteners that it contains can also cause gas. When food reaches the stomach and duodenum, the chemical reactions that are associated with the process of digestion lead to the production of large amounts of gas. The bacteria in the gut can also generate gas especially when they are fermenting fibre that has not been digested by the small bowel. It is, therefore, quite surprising that we only pass wind (flatus) somewhere between five and fifteen times a day. This is because a lot of it is absorbed into the bloodstream and then reaches the lungs where it is released into the breath. Flatus nearly always has some smell attached to it and this is usually worse when the stools are loose. Smell can be affected by certain foods, such as cabbage or sprouts, which can also affect the amount of gas that we pass. Table 2 lists the foods that are more likely to lead to gas.

---

**Table 2** Foods that tend to produce a lot of gas

- Broccoli
- Cabbage
- Brussels Sprouts
- Cauliflower

- Beans
- Onions
- Apples
- Pears
- Prunes
- High-fibre foods such as wholegrain cereals
- Artificial sweeteners
- Chewing gum

---

People vary in their response to gas producing foods so it is up to you to pinpoint the worst offenders for you.

## The brain and the gut

Let's briefly look again at the enteric nervous system (the gut brain). The fact that we feel 'butterflies' in our stomach when we are nervous shows that there must be a strong connection between our brain (central nervous system) and our gut. This is made possible through nerves directly connected to the gut or through hormones released from the brain (neuropeptides) which can then act on the gut. The enteric nervous system allows the gut to function on its own most of the time. However, our brain can override the enteric nervous system under certain circumstances in a positive or negative way. For instance, we can defer bowel opening if it is inconvenient or our tummy can become upset if we are nervous. This connection between gut and brain (the gut–brain axis) can be very important in the understanding of gut disorders, as well as their treatment, as we will see later.

## The bacteria of the gut

The gut microbiome (or microbiota) is the term used to describe the bacteria that live in our gut. The contents of the stomach are relatively germ free because the acid the stomach makes is very good at killing bacteria. However, as things move down the small bowel, progressively more bacteria start to be found until the colon is reached where there is a dramatic increase in their number.

There are millions and millions of bacteria in our colon and it is now becoming recognised that, rather than just being part of the waste material that our body makes, they are actually absolutely essential for our good health. For instance, animals grown in completely germ-free conditions are very unhealthy because their immune system does not develop properly. In addition, we now know that some of the bacteria in our gut can actually reduce our chances of getting gastrointestinal infections. There is even evidence that the make-up of the gut microbiome can influence the activity of the central nervous system which in turn can have an effect on the gut bacteria. Consequently, we need to seriously consider treating the gut bacteria with far more respect than we have in the past. For instance, although antibiotics (which kill bacteria) can be life-saving when we are infected with a dangerous bacteria (pathogens or pathogenic bacteria), they can also kill good bacteria (probiotic bacteria) which is not such a good thing. As we will see later, there is some evidence to suggest that people who, in the past, have taken antibiotics on a long-term basis are more likely to subsequently develop tummy problems.

# CHAPTER 2
# THE ABNORMAL GUT

Just like any other system in the body, the gastrointestinal system (the gut) can start to function abnormally or become diseased. When the problem affects the structure of the gut, such as an ulcer (a break in the lining of the gut), a cancer (a tumour) or inflammation (such as Crohn's disease), it is often referred to as an organic disease. However, when there is no obvious structural abnormality, it is usually referred to as a functional gastrointestinal disorder and IBS is the most common example.

In other words, the gut is not functioning properly, but the tests do not show anything because they are only designed to detect organic problems. This can lead to a major misunderstanding between the patient with tummy problems and their doctor if the patient is told that all the tests are 'normal', sometimes with the implication that 'there is nothing wrong with you'. Unfortunately, we do not have any tests that prove someone has a condition such as IBS, but that does not mean that it does not exist. Hopefully, things will change in the future but, until such a time arrives, patients and, possibly more importantly, doctors have to accept that the diagnosis has to be based on what the patient tells the doctor (a clinical diagnosis) rather than relying on a test. This is not an uncommon problem in other areas of medicine, a good example being migraine. If a person with severe migraine had a computerised tomography (CT) scan of their head during an attack, the scan would be completely 'normal'. However, it would be a very brave doctor who would tell that person that they hadn't got a headache.

## Functional gastrointestinal disorders

A functional gastrointestinal disorder can affect any part of the gastrointestinal system and symptoms can vary depending on which part is involved. Consequently, a person might experience chest pain if the oesophagus (gullet) is involved and, perhaps, nausea or vomiting if the stomach is not working properly. These conditions are given names according to the area affected, with the most common being non-cardiac chest pain (which affects the oesophagus), functional dyspepsia (stomach) and IBS (small and large bowel). However, it is important to recognise that there can be considerable overlap between these conditions and, therefore, some IBS sufferers may, for instance, experience chest pain.

## What causes IBS?

Irritable bowel syndrome is the most common functional gastrointestinal disorder and is the focus of this book. However, it is probable that all the other functional gastrointestinal disorders are caused by similar abnormalities. It is now recognised that there is not a single cause of IBS and that a variety of factors can conspire to bring about symptoms. The technical term for this is a multifactorial disorder. The factors that can bring about IBS are shown in Table 3.

---

**Table 3** Factors contributing to the development of IBS

- Genetic predisposition
- Oversensitivity of the gut (hypersensitivity)
- Muscular overactivity of the gut (dysmotility)
- Abnormal processing of pain signals from the gut by the brain (central processing)
- Disturbance of the balance of the bacteria in the gut (dysbiosis)
- Diet
- Psychological influences

---

## Genetics

There is no doubt that IBS runs in families which suggests that there is a genetic component. However, it is probably not strong enough to make it certain that a particular individual will definitely develop IBS, but means that they might develop it if they happen to be unfortunate enough to be exposed to a particular trigger. We certainly don't know all the possible triggers, although excessive antibiotic usage, particularly in childhood (such as for recurrent tonsillitis) or in adolescence (for something like acne), can cause problems later on. Gastroenteritis is another trigger in some people where it is thought to leave a low-grade inflammation in the gut. Anti-inflammatory drugs, such as ibuprofen, can cause problems and severe stress can also act as a trigger.

When questioned closely a patient with IBS will often say they have always had a mildly sensitive tummy or a slightly irregular bowel habit, but never taken much notice of it. Then, at a certain time, they developed all the symptoms of IBS which became much more troublesome. This particular story of longstanding 'subclinical' symptoms suggests a genetic pre-disposition which is followed by a trigger, which then leads to more severe symptoms recognisable as IBS. This trigger may be obvious in some people, such as an episode of gastroenteri-tis, but not others.

## Hypersensitivity

What actually causes symptoms is gradually beginning to be understood. We now know that the lining of the gut is more sensitive than it should be in IBS (hypersensitivity). This results in people being able to feel their guts, and what is going on in them, more than normal. For instance, a person who does not have IBS only feels what is going on in their rectum when there is enough stool in there to make them want to open their bowels. In contrast, many people with IBS can feel even a tiny piece of stool in their rectum (which there always is) and they, therefore, constantly feel that they want to open their bowels, even though there is not enough to pass. You need a certain volume of stool in your rectum before you are able to push it out.

Similarly, a person with IBS may also have a hypersensitive oesophagus and, if they do, they may experience heartburn (acid in the oesophagus or gullet) with a relatively small amount of acid which would not cause symptoms if the oesophagus was not hypersensitive. At this point, it is important to realise that this hypersensitivity is a real abnormality and it is not just the person being hypersensitive about everything.

## Muscular overactivity

The tummy pain that is experienced by people with IBS is usually due to the contraction (spasm) of the muscles of the bowel and this is sometimes called colic. In the same way that a muscle in your leg can go into spasm and cause a cramp, the muscle of the bowel can do the same. Similarly, it can be mild or very severe and women with IBS often say it is rather like the pains associated with childbirth or sometimes even worse. In addition, the hypersensitivity of the gut can amplify this pain associated with spasm. Pain from the gut can occur in any part of the abdomen but the sufferer will usually be able to say that it is in one general area, although it may not always be limited to that area. The muscles of the anus can also go into spasm leading to very severe pain in the anus which is called proctalgia fugax. Fortunately, this pain doesn't usually last very long as some people say it can be almost unbearable. As the muscular activity of the gut is somewhat disturbed in IBS, it is sometimes referred to as a motility disorder.

## IBS and the nervous system

Obviously, the way we react to pain is controlled by our central nervous system, which is the name given to the brain and spinal cord. The spinal cord has mechanisms for blocking most of the signals coming from our body, otherwise the brain would become overloaded with information. In some conditions, such as IBS, this filter is not quite so efficient and pain signals that may not be so important can get through, which then puts the brain on alert.

Consequently, it is useful to think of IBS as a condition where the gut is 'oversensitive' and 'overreactive'. Therefore, something that would upset the tummy of a person without IBS for a day or two will upset an IBS gut for a week or two.

For instance, this could be a dietary indiscretion, an infection, a side-effect of a medication or a stressful event.

Irritable bowel syndrome has a name for being a largely psychological condition and nothing could be further from the truth. All of us have had experiences where stress affects the gut, such as a sensation of butterflies in the tummy. Consequently, it is not surprising that if someone has an overreactive gut, it is likely to react somewhat more than one that is not hypersensitive. As we will see later, the symptoms of IBS can, in some people, be very severe and this is likely to affect them psychologically. Consequently, when an IBS sufferer appears to have psychological problems, it is important to consider that this may be because of their IBS rather than being the cause of the IBS.

The problem is that as IBS becomes more severe, not surprisingly, a person becomes more and more worried about it. This can then lead to them regularly checking their tummy to see if they have the pain and this can then make them more aware of the problem. This is called hypervigilance and there is evidence that eventually the area in the brain which determines how we react emotionally to pain can become overactive in IBS.

## IBS and bacteria

As we have already seen in Chapter 1, the bacteria in the gut (the microbiome) play a very important role in maintaining health. It is, therefore, not surprising that, if the balance between the millions of bacteria is disturbed, this might have consequences for our health.

There are several reasons why this could happen in IBS. Firstly, having gastroenteritis or taking antibiotics can profoundly affect the make-up of the microbiome. Secondly, various dietary constituents can encourage, or discourage, the growth of bacteria. Certain carbohydrates are particularly effective at promoting the growth of good bacteria and are often referred to as prebiotics. Lastly, if the motility (see page 11) of the gut is disturbed, this can affect the flow through the gut which can then influence the growth of bacteria. Just like a blocked or slow-running drain which becomes smelly because of an accumulation of bacteria, a gut that is not working properly can run into problems with overgrowth of bacteria. When this occurs in the small bowel (small intestine), it is often called small intestinal bacterial overgrowth (SIBO) and this issue is now receiving a lot of attention (see page 116). However, we are not sure whether the SIBO causes the symptoms or is just a result of the motility problem. Obviously, if it is just the result of a motility problem, then treating it may not be particularly helpful as it will return unless something can be done about the motility problem itself.

## IBS and diet

Irritable bowel syndrome sufferers often say that eating makes their symptoms worse. Consequently, they often think that they have some form of dietary allergy or intolerance. In fact, dietary allergy is rather uncommon in IBS, but many sufferers are intolerant of certain foods and excluding such foods can be a very useful treatment option (see Chapter 5).

## Putting it all together

It is likely that a person must have a susceptibility to IBS in the first place, probably genetic, before they can develop the condition. It is also more likely that different factors are more important in different people and the 'dose' of these factors is critical. Consequently, if the 'dose' of a particular factor is very high it may almost be able to trigger the problem on its own without the need for any other activating factors.

One way of thinking about this is by using a point system. For instance, if you need 100 points to get symptoms, then if diet is putting in 70, you have only got 30 left for other things. Consequently, if stress is putting in 40 you are in trouble, but if on another day stress is only putting in 20 points then you will be okay. This example is only using two factors and in reality, as we have already seen, there are far more than just two, which makes things more complicated. However, we can do more about some factors than others and, therefore, these are the ones we should be targeting with treatment. For instance, as we will see later, a bowl of bran is probably worth nearly 100 points whereas a portion of carrots amounts to only a couple of points, giving us an opportunity to reduce the input of points from the diet. This then leaves us with more points to accommodate factors we can do less about, such as stress or the menstrual cycle in women. In addition, some of the medications used in IBS might decrease the number of points by reducing the hypersensitivity of the bowel (see chapter 7). Unfortunately, the importance of the different triggers varies considerably from person to person. Therefore, two IBS sufferers with identical symptoms may respond completely differently to a particular treatment depending on what factors are 'driving' their symptoms. At the present time there is no sure way of determining which factors are important in a particular person, so the approach to treatment often has to be by 'trial and error'.

# CHAPTER 3
# SYMPTOMS OF IBS

The principal symptoms of IBS are abdominal pain, an abnormal bowel habit and abdominal bloating. However, as we shall see later, people with IBS frequently suffer from a whole range of other 'non-colonic' symptoms which can cause lots of problems and are not always recognised by the medical profession.

## Abdominal pain

The pain can be felt in any part of the abdomen but is most common on the left-hand side. In some people the pain can occur in different places at different times and, in others, the whole abdomen can be affected. Most people describe the pain as stabbing, twisting or squeezing, although some say it is just a dull ache. The severity of the pain can vary from day to day but sometimes it can be so strong that sufferers say they can't stand up straight or have to curl up in a ball. Women often say the pain can be as bad, or even worse, than that which they experienced during childbirth. Many of them say 'surely there must be something really serious going on with pain as bad as this'. It is also very distressing for relatives or partners to see someone in such pain as they feel so helpless and, occasionally, the pain can be so bad that the IBS sufferer has to go to the A&E department.

It is important to realise that, however severe the pain might be, it is not damaging your gut in any way and it will eventually improve. The gut cannot stay in severe spasm forever but, just like when you do some activity or exercise that you are not used to, the muscles can ache and remain tender for quite a long time after the severe spasm has subsided. Some people even say that their tummy is always rather tender to the extent that they have to be careful about putting too much pressure on it.

## Abnormal bowel habit

The bowel habit in IBS can take the form of diarrhoea or constipation and, in some people, it fluctuates between these two extremes. In people with diarrhoea, the stools can vary from just being soft through to a consistency of porridge or even water. Sufferers often have to rush to the toilet and can even have 'accidents' with their bowels. Even one accident is a disaster and when they occur frequently it is devastating and it is difficult to talk about this side of the problem. We have found that a quarter of IBS patients attending our clinic have not told anyone about their incontinence and half have not informed their general practitioner about this problem.

It is soul-destroying to have to carry a change of clothing or wear incontinence pads and you would be surprised if you knew just how many IBS sufferers have to do this. In addition, when a sufferer goes out, they need to know the location of all the toilets in the place they are visiting. This can be a particular problem when they are going to an unfamiliar area or in certain situations, such as getting stuck in traffic. A particularly frustrating aspect of the problem is its unpredictability. A person with IBS never knows when the problem is going to strike next and, when it does, it can be completely out of the blue. In some people the diarrhoea can be on a continuous basis and in some instances these people become housebound.

Another major problem is that the diarrhoea can be made worse by eating because of the exaggerated gastrocolonic response (see page 14). Consequently, instead of just wanting to open their bowels after breakfast, many people with IBS need to go to the toilet after every meal because this gastrocolonic response lasts all day rather than just being present in the morning. In addition, eating can bring on their pain. This can make people afraid to go out to restaurants or visit their friends. Even when they have been to the toilet, their bowels never feel empty because of the hypersensitivity (see page 22). Not surprisingly, some people get a very sore bottom, which is a common problem in any form of diarrhoea. The diarrhoea associated with IBS is largely due to rapid movement through the colon rather than the small bowel and, therefore, food, nutrients and medication are usually absorbed normally. This helps to explain why people with diarrhoea-type IBS do not necessarily lose weight, as the small bowel has absorbed their food normally.

In constipation, the stools can be hard, pellety (like rabbit droppings), stringy and can sometimes be flat or curved. People often have difficulty pushing out their stools and can have to strain for long periods of time. Even if they do manage to go, they seldom feel empty, which again is due to the hypersensitivity. The frequency of going to the toilet in constipation can vary enormously. Even if someone goes to the toilet every day but has to struggle to pass a very hard stool, they should be considered to be constipated. It goes without saying that, if someone goes for many days without a bowel movement, they are constipated. Some people can go for a week or even longer without a successful bowel movement. This can lead to other symptoms such as headaches and bad breath and some people say that they almost feel they are being 'poisoned' by all the faeces building up inside them.

Constipation can be due to two main causes. These are, firstly, a problem with the propulsion of faeces through the colon or, secondly, a problem with the actual mechanism for expelling the faeces (defaecation). The process of defaecation is actually quite complicated and involves the relaxation of the anal sphincter (see page 12) and also relaxation of an internal muscle (the puborectalis) that normally keeps the rectum at an angle to help preserve continence. For reasons that are unknown, some people with IBS actually contract their anal sphincter and the puborectalis when they try to open their bowels and are obviously pushing against a closed door. This condition is called obstructed defaecation or anismus. It is important to try and recognise these two different types of constipation, as the propulsion problem responds better to laxatives than anismus, which often does better with biofeedback (see page 107).

When constipation sufferers do manage to go, their stool can be so hard that it splits their anus, which can cause pain and bleeding – this is called an anal fissure. Another problem that can occur as a result of straining is the development of haemorrhoids (piles) which are enlarged veins similar to varicose veins which can bleed and feel like soft lumps under the skin of the anus. Sometimes, someone can develop a hard lump under the skin which is very painful and is dark blue or purple in colour. This is due to a hard stool causing bleeding under the skin, rather like a blood blister. The medical term for this problem is a peri-anal haematoma and these can take a few weeks to settle down. Occasionally, if the left side of a person's colon is sufficiently 'loaded' with constipated faeces, they can actually feel a lumpy colon with their hand. Not surprisingly, this can be very alarming if they don't know what they are feeling, but it is nothing to worry about. However, it does mean that they should be treating their constipation, as we will see later. Faecal incontinence can also be a problem in constipation-type IBS, either because of laxatives or because the colon suddenly decides to empty itself without warning.

Some constipated people can develop what is called overflow diarrhoea, sometimes referred to as spurious diarrhoea. This is where the lower part of the bowel is blocked with hard stool which only allows liquid and mucus to pass around it, giving the impression of diarrhoea. It is very important to recognise this problem, otherwise a doctor might recommend an antidiarrhoea medication which will make the situation worse. This problem can usually be identified by a doctor examining the tummy and rectum, but if there is uncertainty a simple X-ray can confirm the diagnosis.

Needless to say, someone who has a bowel habit that alternates between constipation and diarrhoea can suffer from all of the problems that can occur with both diarrhoea or constipation and this can be particularly hard to treat. However, it is important to realise that if someone with diarrhoea medication on an intermittent basis or a constipation sufferer uses their laxative irregularly, this can lead to an apparently alternating bowel habit. This is why when taking laxatives or antidiarrhoea medications it is better to take a low dose on a regular basis rather than intermittent large doses. Obviously, if someone has a truly alternating bowel habit then they have no option other than

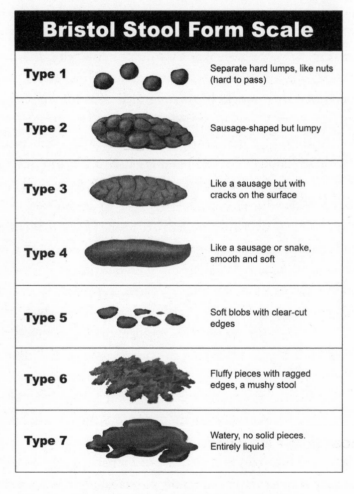

Figure 2 The Bristol Stool Form Scale

to use both laxatives and antidiarrhoea medication as judiciously as possible.

Many people find it very embarrassing to talk about their stools, especially when they are asked to describe them. The Bristol Stool Form Scale (Figure 2) is a useful way of overcoming this problem as people can then just point to the relative picture or say the number (types 1–7) that is beside the picture. It is important to realise that stool form can vary from day to day and some people will pass a variety of forms in one bowel opening.

## Incomplete evacuation

As we have already seen, a feeling of incomplete emptying of the rectum is extremely common in IBS. This results in people repetitively visiting the toilet and straining to empty their bowel, usually with little success. The cause of this problem is hypersensitivity of the rectum which leads the brain to think there is stool in the rectum that needs to be expelled when, actually, there is not enough to pass. Consequently, it is important to try to resist the temptation to keep on trying to open the bowels, as the straining can lead to stretching of the rectum which can actually make the bowel even more sensitive. Therefore, if you feel you have passed enough stool for one day, it is advisable to try and ignore this symptom, although that is easier said than done.

## Bloating and distension

Bloating is an extremely common and troublesome symptom of IBS. In some people the tummy just feels swollen but, in others, it can actually swell up and some women can look as if they are in the late stages of pregnancy. This is called abdominal distension (see Figure 3).

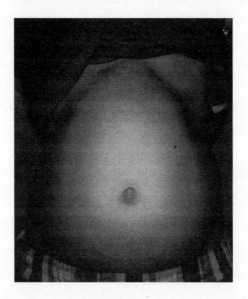

Figure 3 A young female with severe abdominal distension due to IBS

Although bloating and distension can occur at any time, they are least troublesome in the morning and gradually get worse during the day. By the end of the day sufferers often have to loosen their clothing or even change into a different size of clothing. Not surprisingly, people with IBS find this problem very distressing and some say it is their most intrusive symptom. Abdominal distension can put pressure on the bladder that can lead to the desire to pass urine frequently and the distension may even make some people feel breathless.

The cause of distension is very complicated but it is not usually due to excess gas. It seems to be more related to the fact that the diaphragm (a muscle that helps you to breathe) doesn't contract and relax normally, which explains why some people with distension also feel breathless. Bloating and distension can also make heartburn worse because the increased pressure aggravates any tendency towards acid reflux.

Bloating and distension seem to be more common in women but this is partly because men describe this problem differently. They often say their tummy feels tight or hard rather than necessarily looking distended. This may be because the abdominal muscles of men tend to be stronger and obviously are not designed to allow for the accommodation of the pregnant uterus.

A very important point to remember is that if you have abdominal distension that does not go up and down during the course of the day, you should always have this investigated further in case it is not related to IBS. There are plenty of people with IBS who have persistent distension, but it is best to get it checked before assuming it is due to IBS.

## Gas

As we have already seen (see page 16), we all produce a certain amount of gas on a daily basis. However, because of the hypersensitivity of the gut in IBS, sufferers develop more gas-related symptoms which can be extremely intrusive, especially if the wind has an offensive smell. It goes without saying, this can affect a person's life in a whole variety of ways and we see women who are even reluctant to have relationships because of this problem.

## Borborygmi

Borborygmi is the technical term for the noises or rumbling that any tummy can make and is a reflection of the normal muscular activity of the gut. Not surprisingly, in IBS these noises can be much louder because the muscular activity of the gut is so much more vigorous in this condition. Some people say their gut is so active that they can feel all of this going on inside them, whereas people without IBS can't usually feel anything. This problem can be very embarrassing especially for people who work with others in particularly quiet environments.

## The non-colonic symptoms of IBS

The non-colonic symptoms of IBS are listed in Table 4 (page 39) and include low back pain, constant lethargy or tiredness, thigh pain (in one or both legs), nausea (and occasionally vomiting), bladder symptoms, headaches, chest pain and pain on intercourse in women.

The bladder symptoms represent an irritable bladder which is quite common in IBS and can include frequency, urgency and, in men, difficulty passing urine. These bladder symptoms can make doctors think they are dealing with cystitis and offer antibiotics. In IBS antibiotics should only be given if the urine tests positive for infection, as antibiotics can make IBS worse.

Irritable bowel syndrome can have a huge impact on sexual activity, especially in women. Pain with intercourse is quite common and can even come on after sex and go on for several days afterwards. Also, intercourse can put pressure on the bowel with obvious consequences. If the woman also has bladder symptoms such as frequency or urgency due to an irritable bladder, this makes things even more difficult. Lastly, sex can be affected by the psychological consequences of all these problems, not to mention the negative effect that a problem such as abdominal distension or faecal incontinence can have on body image.

Feeling constantly tired and lethargic is very demoralising, especially if it is coupled with nausea and headaches. The low backache raises the possibility of arthritis of the spine or a disc problem, especially in somebody over the age of 50, when some degree of spinal arthritis is quite common. However, it is important to sort out what is actually causing the pain and to avoid arthritis medications, if possible, as they often upset IBS.

It is very important that doctors recognise these non-colonic features as otherwise they may refer the sufferer to the wrong specialist and that can lead to inappropriate treatment. For instance, it has been shown that people with IBS are seen in gynaecological, bladder or even chest pain clinics, where they don't do well because they don't have the problem in which the clinic specialises. Sometimes, the chest pain can be such a problem that sufferers go to the A&E department because they think they may be having a heart attack. Of course, it is very important that, for example, a heart problem is not missed by doing the necessary tests. However, once the tests have been completed and if there is also an abnormal bowel habit, tummy pain and bloating, the possibility of IBS causing the chest pain needs to be seriously considered.

With all the various symptoms that people with IBS report to their doctor, it is perhaps not surprising that doctors are puzzled about how to treat them or whom to refer them to. For instance, if the pain is near where the appendix or gall bladder are located (see Figure 1 on page 7), then there may be the temptation to remove that particular organ. Similarly, if a woman with IBS has a scan of her tummy and is found to have an ovarian cyst, which may actually be painless, then if the pain from the IBS is near the location of the cyst, the question of removing the cyst arises. Obviously a large ovarian cyst needs to be taken seriously but many cysts are quite small and can actually disappear over time. Now that scans (ultrasound, CT or MRI scans) are done so often, ovarian cysts are frequently found and, as long as they are not large or suspected of being malignant, they should probably be observed rather than removed in someone with IBS.

Another condition that can be found on a scan is polycystic ovary syndrome (PCOS). This is a condition where the ovaries contain multiple cysts and can be associated with a tendency to be overweight. It does not seem to be related to IBS and, if it is found in someone with IBS symptoms, is very unlikely to be the cause of all their tummy symptoms.

Having knowledge of these difficult situations puts you in a position to be able to discuss the options with your doctor so that it is more likely that the right decision is made. It is awful to have an operation that it is hoped will get rid of the pain only to find that it has not helped at all. To make matters worse, surgery on the tummy in IBS does tend to escalate the IBS symptoms so that is another reason to avoid surgery, if at all possible. If something is found that is unlikely to be causing the IBS symptoms and is safe to ignore for a while, it is much better to treat the IBS first. If the symptoms persist, then the situation can always be reconsidered at a later date.

Some people say that their non-colonic symptoms cause more trouble than their bowel symptoms. We always ask a person with IBS to name their worst symptom or, if they could only get rid of one symptom, which one would they choose. This is very useful in guiding treatment as it is not always, as many doctors think, the abdominal pain that a person finds to be the most intrusive. For instance, some patients might say it is the bloating or the constant lethargy that bothers them most and, for women, the pain on intercourse can be a major problem.

---

**Table 4** Non-colonic symptoms of IBS

- Constant lethargy or tiredness*
- Low backache*
- Nausea, usually without vomiting*
- Bladder symptoms*
- Headaches
- Chest pain
- Thigh pain in one or both legs
- Pain on intercourse in women
- Joint pains

* These are the most common symptoms associated with IBS

---

## Fibromyalgia

Fibromyalgia is the name given to a condition where the joints become tender and painful and it can develop in people with IBS. This problem is different to arthritis, where the joints become inflamed which can lead to them becoming damaged over time. The good news about fibromyalgia is that the joints do not become damaged however long you have the condition. The cause of fibromyalgia is not exactly known, but it is likely that the joints have become 'oversensitive' in some way rather like the gut is oversensitive in IBS.

## Other symptoms

Some people with IBS say they get a temperature when their IBS flares up, but if they took their temperature during a flare-up, they would find it to be normal. This problem is caused by the autonomic nervous system (see page 13) being overactive in some IBS sufferers which can also lead to other symptoms such as excessive sweating, palpitations and, if the blood pressure drops, feeling faint. Consequently, if you think you are getting a temperature, you should check it with a thermometer and it should be normal. Irritable bowel syndrome does not cause a raised temperature.

## The menstrual cycle

Many women without any gastrointestinal problems at all notice that their bowel function may change slightly around the time of their periods. Therefore, it comes as no great surprise that IBS symptoms can get worse at the time of menstruation. This is a very important observation as it can lead both the IBS sufferer and their doctor to wrongly conclude that the problem is gynaecological in origin. Therefore, just because IBS symptoms get worse with periods, it does not necessarily mean there is a gynaecological problem, although the possibility has to be borne in mind. When this issue is particularly severe, it can sometimes be helped by suppressing the periods by either taking the pill on a continuous basis for a while or trying a Mirena coil.

## Ovarian cancer

Many women with IBS worry about the possibility of ovarian cancer, although this form of cancer is not more common in women with IBS. However, sufferers feel that, because they have a variety of tummy-related symptoms, something like ovarian cancer could be overlooked. If you are concerned about this issue, then this form of cancer can easily be screened for with either a simple ultrasound scan of the tummy or a blood test called a CA125, or a combination of the two.

## Medications causing gastrointestinal symptoms

A wide range of medications can cause gastrointestinal symptoms in people without gastrointestinal problems and these can be more pronounced in IBS. It is, therefore, always important to check what medications a particular person with IBS is taking, as it is illogical to treat a person with medication for a symptom that is being caused or made worse by another medication.

A wide range of symptoms can be caused by certain medications and these include diarrhoea, constipation, nausea, abdominal pain and bloating. Painkillers (analgesics) are one of the worst offenders – as every one of them, except paracetamol and anti-inflammatory analgesics, can cause constipation. However, the anti-inflammatory analgesics can upset IBS in other ways and should be avoided in this condition if at all possible. If someone with IBS needs an analgesic for any reason, the best choice is paracetamol although it has to be acknowledged that alternatives such as codeine have better analgesic activity. Proton pump inhibitors such as omeprazole, which are frequently used to treat heartburn, can cause diarrhoea and some people find statins (which are taken to lower cholesterol) hard to tolerate. Other medications that can cause problems are iron preparations and metformin, which is mainly used in diabetes.

## Eating disorders

As we have already seen, many people with IBS find that eating makes their symptoms worse, to the extent that some sufferers even say that if they didn't have to eat they would be fine. Not surprisingly, some find it easier to not eat very much with resulting weight loss and then are mistakenly diagnosed as having an eating disorder. Obviously, if an IBS sufferer does have a real eating disorder as well as their IBS, this is a really problematic combination of conditions, which can be extremely difficult to treat.

## Psychological symptoms

People with IBS may suffer from psychological symptoms such as anxiety, which has resulted in some members of the medical profession claiming that IBS is a psychological condition. However, if those doctors themselves had all the symptoms that we have been talking about in this chapter, it seems likely that they would also become anxious. Consequently, it is unfair to label IBS as a psychosomatic condition as the symptoms are just as real as for any other disorder. The only psychological feature that does seem to be quite common in IBS sufferers is a tendency to be a bit of a worrier, but even that could be as a result of their illness.

It is important to remember that there is a strong connection between the brain and the gut which is sometimes called 'the gut–brain axis' (see page 17). Even people without any bowel problems at all will notice some gastrointestinal symptoms before, for instance, public speaking. Consequently, it would be rather surprising if stress did not make the gut in IBS a little more irritable, but that doesn't mean that stress is the cause. However, if a person does have some significant psychological problems these will make their IBS symptoms worse, but any disease is made worse by psychological distress.

## Relationships

Irritable bowel syndrome can have a profound impact on relationships. Sufferers can become very nervous about going out of their comfort zone and, therefore, often shy away from socialising, eating out, travelling or going on holiday. Not surprisingly, partners can become very frustrated by this especially if they are wrongly under the impression that IBS is 'all in the head' and their partner just needs to 'pull themself together'. To make matters worse, sexual function can be affected in sufferers of both sexes. In women, intercourse can be painful and there may be the fear of passing wind or even worse during sex. In addition, if they are very bloated they feel less attractive. In men, sex drive can become much reduced and having sex can also make their symptoms worse. We find that seeing the patient and their partner together can be very helpful so that we can educate the partner about IBS and how it can affect people as well as assuring them that the sufferer has a completely legitimate illness.

## IBS in Crohn's disease and ulcerative colitis

Crohn's disease and ulcerative colitis, collectively known as inflammatory bowel disease (IBD), are inflammatory conditions of the gut that are completely different and separate from IBS. Although Crohn's disease and ulcerative colitis are usually regarded by doctors as being more serious than IBS, there are actually far more effective treatments available for them than IBS. In addition, the quality of life of people with severe IBS can be much worse than that of people with IBD. There is no evidence that IBS predisposes people to IBD. As we have already seen (see page 21), any type of inflammatory process, such as viral or bacterial gastroenteritis, can trigger IBS in a susceptible person. It is, therefore, not surprising that the inflammation in IBD can also lead to these patients developing IBS. Consequently, if a person with IBD continues to get symptoms despite their inflammation being under complete control, it is important that their doctors consider the possibility that their symptoms might be due to IBS.

Occasionally, people get confused by the abbreviations IBS and IBD as they are so similar, especially as doctors use them frequently rather than using the complete terms irritable bowel syndrome and inflammatory bowel disease. They are completely different conditions requiring completely different treatment, although some unlucky people with IBD can develop IBS when their IBD is in remission.

## CHAPTER 4
# THE DIAGNOSIS OF IBS

The diagnosis of IBS is what is called a 'clinical diagnosis'. This means that the doctor has to make the diagnosis based on the symptoms that you, the sufferer, describe to him or her. Unfortunately, there is no test that can confirm the diagnosis and the only reason for doing tests is to rule out any other condition that might be giving similar symptoms.

As we have already seen, the main symptoms of IBS are abdominal (tummy) pain or discomfort, an abnormal bowel habit (constipation, diarrhoea or an alternation between the two patterns) and abdominal bloating which may be a feeling of pressure in the tummy or an actual increase in its size (distension), which can look like pregnancy. When someone suffers from these symptoms, it is very likely that they have IBS. In addition, IBS very commonly runs in families, suggesting a genetic component, so if you have a relative with IBS, your symptoms are more likely to be due to IBS. If someone with gastrointestinal symptoms also has some or all of the non-colonic symptoms that were mentioned in the previous chapter, then this makes the diagnosis of IBS very likely.

After a doctor has gone through all the symptoms and they are consistent with IBS, a 'positive' diagnosis should be made although other possibilities may have to be considered and, if necessary, ruled out with the appropriate tests. For instance, if a person is over the age of 50 it is sensible to rule out the possibility of bowel (colon) cancer, although the symptoms of bowel cancer seldom mimic those of IBS. The worst start for someone with IBS is to be submitted to a whole battery of tests and then be told that they are all normal and there is nothing wrong with them, so it is probably IBS. That is a very 'negative' way of making the diagnosis and leaves the patient thinking that the doctor is just calling it IBS because they don't really know what is wrong with the patient. This can make some sufferers think that something is being missed and this is a problem because, as long as someone doesn't believe the diagnosis, it is virtually impossible to move forward with treatment.

## Abdominal pain

The pain in IBS is usually squeezing or twisting (colicky, like a spasm) and some women say it is rather similar to labour pains. It can last a variable length of time and some people have it all the time while in others it can be intermittent. It varies in severity but it can be so intense that the sufferer cannot stand up straight or has to curl up in a ball. It can occur in any part of the abdomen and Figure 4 shows the various areas where pain can be felt and the medical words that are used to describe these areas. It most commonly occurs in areas 6 and 9 but can be felt in any other region or all over the tummy. Unfortunately, when it happens in some areas, other possible causes have to be considered.

Many IBS sufferers feel hot and sweaty when they get an attack of pain and assume they have got a temperature. Irritable bowel syndrome never causes a temperature and

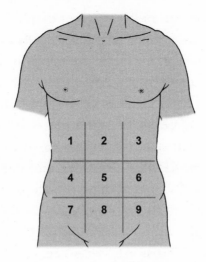

1   Right hypochondrium (pain in this region is called right hypochondrial pain)
2   Epigastrium (pain in this region is called epigastric pain)
3   Left hypochondrium
4   Right lumbar region
5   Umbilical region (pain in this region is often called central abdominal pain)
6   Left lumbar region
7   Right iliac fossa (pain in this region is called right iliac fossa pain)
8   Hypogastrium or suprapubic region
9   Left iliac fossa

Figure 4 The names given to the various
regions of the abdomen

we advise our patients to buy a thermometer so that they
can check their temperature in such circumstances. It is
nearly always normal but, if it isn't, then further investigation is always necessary.

Area 1 in Figure 4 is called the right hypochondrium and
the gall bladder is located inside the abdomen in this region.
Consequently, pain in this area raises the possibility of gall
bladder problems such as gallstones and an ultrasound scan

should be done. The problem is that even if gallstones are found they may be 'silent' and not actually causing symptoms. It is important that the doctor questions you carefully to try and detect some of the differences that can sometimes, but not always, help to separate the two conditions. The main symptom of gall bladder problems is intermittent pain in the right hypochondrium which can go through to the right shoulder blade. This is often accompanied by intolerance of fatty foods and episodes of quite severe vomiting. The tummy can be tender in this area but that can also happen in IBS. If, in addition to gallstones, the gall bladder is inflamed then there may be a temperature and then you can be sure it is not IBS. In this situation the pain is usually continuous rather than intermittent. An ultrasound examination is good at identifying the difference between uncomplicated gallstones and gallstones in conjunction with an inflamed gall bladder. Occasionally, the only way to know for sure that the gall bladder is the source of the problem is to remove it, a procedure called a cholecystectomy. However, this is a risky strategy as not only will the pain persist if the gall bladder was not the cause of the problem, but surgery can sometimes make the pain worse. Therefore, if you are ever in this situation it is important that you have a very frank conversation with the surgeon to make sure they are not just removing the gall bladder in case it is the cause. Another important point is that, if you have your gall bladder removed, this can lead to diarrhoea, so people with IBS need to be aware of this potential problem, especially if they have the diarrhoea version of IBS.

If the pain is in area 7, which is called the right iliac fossa, then the appendix may come under suspicion. Appendicitis is usually quite easy to separate from IBS as the infection leads to a temperature and also results in some abnormal blood tests called inflammatory markers – a high white blood cell count and a raised C-reactive protein (CRP). A high white blood cell count and CRP tells you there is inflammation in the body but does not tell you where it is, so you have to do more tests to find the location of the inflammation. The tummy is extremely tender in appendicitis and an ultrasound examination confirms the diagnosis. In someone who keeps getting pain in the right iliac fossa with no other abnormalities it is important to avoid surgery as, not only will an operation not cure the pain, it could make it worse. In the past, people with continuing pain in the right iliac fossa have been told they may have chronic appendicitis and been offered surgery. If the appendix is chronically inflamed, it will show up on a scan and, therefore, if the scan is normal, you cannot have chronic appendicitis.

Pain in the left side of the abdomen (area 6 or 9 or both of Figure 4) raises the possibility of diverticulitis. As we get older the colon can develop small pouches in its lining, mainly on the left side and particularly in the sigmoid colon (see Figure 1 on page 7). When this happens it is called diverticular disease – another name for it is diverticulosis. Diverticular disease is a very common condition as we get older and the majority of people don't even know they have got it, as it usually remains completely 'silent' throughout life. The number of pouches varies considerably from the person to another and they only become painful if one or more of them become infected and inflamed which is then called diverticulitis. The symptoms of diverticulitis are completely different to IBS and are similar to appendicitis but on the left side. Consequently, the person has severe pain in areas 6 and 9 of Figure 4, which are very tender, coupled with a temperature and raised inflammatory markers (white blood cell count and CRP). An ultrasound or CT scan is very helpful in confirming the diagnosis. If a person has diverticulitis they definitely need antibiotics but these drugs should be avoided if it is just a flare-up of IBS as, not only are they unnecessary, but they can make the symptoms worse. Remember, if you have IBS and are found to have diverticular disease it is far more likely that the IBS is causing your symptoms rather than anything to do with the diverticular disease. Unfortunately, diverticulitis usually causes pain in areas 6 and 9 which are the very areas where IBS pain commonly occurs. However, if there is extreme tenderness, a temperature and signs of inflammation, then diverticular disease needs to be considered. Consequently, it is very important to know the difference between diverticulitis and diverticular disease as people can become very confused about this problem.

Occasionally, a person with diverticular disease can have so many pouches, particularly in the sigmoid colon, that it can become narrow and cause problems, but this is very unusual. Another problem that can happen with diverticular disease is an episode of quite severe bleeding but this is uncommon and usually occurs in people over the age of 60. It can be alarming as there may be quite a lot of blood. However, when someone passes a lot of bright red blood it is nearly always due to diverticular disease and is virtually never due to anything serious like bowel cancer. Fortunately, this bleeding usually settles down very quickly without any treatment but you should always consult your doctor if it happens.

The lower end of the gullet, stomach and duodenum are situated under area 2 (see Figure 4) and this area is called the epigastrium. When pain is situated in this area (known as epigastric pain) a gastric or duodenal ulcer may be suspected but this is easily sorted out by passing a camera into the stomach and duodenum in a procedure called a gastroscopy. Patients having a gastroscopy are frequently found to have a hiatus hernia which is where a part of the stomach rises above the diaphragm (see page 7). Normally all of the stomach stays below the diaphragm. A hiatus hernia is an extremely common finding and can lead to acid refluxing into the gullet (oesophagus) where it can cause heartburn. However, a hiatus hernia does not cause colicky pain in the epigastrium and this type of pain will be coming from spasm somewhere in the small or large bowel as some of the small and large bowel are located in the epigastrium (see Figure 1 on page 7 and Figure 4).

## An abnormal bowel habit

The normal variation in bowel habit has already been described in Chapter 1. In IBS we see great extremes in bowel function depending on which type of IBS we are dealing with. Someone with diarrhoea-type IBS may go anything between four and twenty times a day with either porridgey or watery stools and the need to use the toilet instantly. Some people even have accidents with their bowels which is obviously devastating. The constipation sufferers may not go for a few days or a couple of weeks and struggle to pass very hard stools with a lot of pain and even some bleeding, if they cut their anus with a very large, hard stool. Many people alternate between these different patterns and others can pass a mixture of stools in one bowel opening, starting off hard and then becoming loose. A lot of people say that after they have opened their bowels, they never feel empty. One of the most frustrating things about IBS is that it is completely unpredictable. Many IBS sufferers say they never know when they are going to have a good day or a bad day with their condition. Some poor sufferers have symptoms all the time.

The bowel symptoms described above strongly suggest IBS and, if there is constipation, investigations are seldom necessary unless there is bleeding. However diarrhoea can be caused by other conditions and should be investigated further. In a young person Crohn's disease or ulcerative colitis need to be considered and there is now quite a good screening test that can be performed on the stools (or faeces) called the faecal calprotectin test. If this is negative, Crohn's disease or ulcerative colitis are extremely unlikely, but if it is not negative, you need a camera passing up into your bowel via the anus and this is called a colonoscopy.

It is always important to consider the possibility of Crohn's disease in someone with suspected IBS and diarrhoea. However, it is usually relatively easy to separate the two conditions based on symptoms and Table 5 lists the more common features of Crohn's disease. Ulcerative colitis also causes diarrhoea but this is nearly always bloodstained, so usually gets sorted out very quickly. If there is any doubt about the possibility of ulcerative colitis or Crohn's disease then these two conditions can be ruled out by doing a CRP, a faecal calprotectin test and a colonoscopy. There are other causes of diarrhoea but the only other important one is coeliac disease.

---

**Table 5** Typical symptoms that can occur in Crohn's disease

- Weight loss
- Diarrhoea often, but not always, with blood in the stools
- Tummy pain
- Mouth ulcers
- Joint pains
- Sore eyes
- Temperature

**Plus**

- Positive blood tests for inflammation (raised CRP and white blood cell count)
- Positive stool test for inflammation (faecal calprotectin)
- Crohn's disease or ulcerative colitis in the family

---

Coeliac disease is a condition where wheat can damage the gut and is extremely common, affecting approximately 1 in 100 of the population. In many people it does not cause symptoms but in the more severe cases it can lead to loose bowels, abdominal bloating, weight loss, mouth ulcers and anaemia. The symptoms can be very similar to IBS but it is easily detected by a blood test, although the diagnosis has to be confirmed by a biopsy taken at the same time as having a gastroscopy. If coeliac disease is confirmed you need to go on a gluten-free diet for the rest of your life as the gluten damages the bowel rather than just causing an intolerance. Coeliac disease seems to make some people more susceptible to IBS and the IBS symptoms can persist even when they are on a gluten-free diet. However, it is still important to continue with the gluten-free diet as continuing to eat gluten will harm the gut. The IBS will also need to be treated in the usual way, as will be discussed later.

A change in bowel habit can be the first symptom of bowel cancer so this is a good opportunity to deal with this issue in order to put it in perspective and stop people worrying about it. Bowel cancer is one of the more common cancers but, unlike some forms of malignancy, it is nearly always curable if detected at an early stage. Consequently, it is very important to look for bowel cancer if there is any suspicion that someone might have this disease. It is uncommon under the age of 50, unless there is a family history of a relative having it under that age, but it becomes more common as you get older.

Bowel cancer does not give the symptoms of IBS and actually can be quite 'silent' initially. One important symptom is rectal bleeding but this is quite common in IBS. It is often relatively easy to identify the cause of bleeding in IBS, especially if someone has piles, a fissure (see page 30), a sore bottom because of diarrhoea or is passing large hard stools. For instance, if the blood drips from the anus it is likely to be due to haemorrhoids or if the bleeding is associated with a sharp tearing sensation it is probably an anal fissure. If an obvious cause cannot be identified then it is best to have the colon examined with a colonoscopy (see page 54) even if you are relatively young, just to be on the safe side.

The other main symptom resulting from bowel cancer is a change in bowel habit. This is usually easy to recognise in someone who doesn't have IBS but people with IBS often ask, 'How would I know as I already have a changed bowel habit?' This is a difficult question to answer but even someone with IBS can often tell that 'something has changed from my usual IBS symptoms'.

It is very important that people with IBS know that IBS does not increase the risk of developing bowel cancer. The government have introduced a screening test for bowel cancer for people over the age of 60. This involves testing a stool sample for traces of blood (the faecal occult blood test) and, if blood is found, then it is necessary to do a colonoscopy. This policy results in quite a lot of people having a normal colonoscopy as not everybody with blood in their stools turns out to have bowel cancer. However, it is quite a good test to detect bowel cancer and if you are worried about this possibility, it would be worth asking your general practitioner to do a faecal occult blood test on a sample of your stools. However, if you have a tendency to rectal bleeding which has been previously investigated, a faecal occult blood test would not be appropriate as it will inevitably be positive. It is likely that in the near future stool tests that check for the presence of cancer DNA will be available and these will obviously be far more accurate than the current practice of testing for occult blood. With regard to IBS, the take-home message is that IBS doesn't cause bowel cancer and the vast majority of people with IBS never develop this disease.

## Bloating

Many people with bloating say that it is their worst symptom (see page 34). In some it is a feeling of pressure in the tummy but in others the abdomen can actually swell alarmingly (as shown in Figure 3 on page 34). The cause is very complicated but it is seldom due to gas and, in many, it is caused by spasm of the diaphragm and that is why some people feel breathless. Bloating and distension are usually least troublesome in the morning and then gradually get worse during the course of the day. If someone describes this pattern of bloating and distension, going up and down over 24 hours, it is absolutely typical for IBS and other related functional gastrointestinal disorders and is not seen in any other condition. It is, therefore, really useful in confirming the diagnosis of IBS. If the abdomen is distended and does not fluctuate, this can happen in very severe IBS, but it can be a clue that something else is going on, such as a gynaecological problem, and should always be investigated.

## Non-colonic symptoms

As already described, people with IBS can experience a range of other symptoms such as low backache, lethargy, nausea, bladder and gynaecological symptoms (see Table 4 on page 39). These are important because, if someone suffers from these symptoms, it makes the diagnosis of IBS more certain. They are also important because they can lead to the doctor investigating them unnecessarily or even sending them to the wrong specialist. For instance, if you are feeling tired all the time, the doctor may keep checking you for anaemia or an underactive thyroid. Alternatively, you may be referred to a bladder specialist if you are suffering from an irritable bladder which is quite common in IBS (see page 36).

## Gynaecological symptoms

As we have already seen (see page 40), women with IBS often suffer from symptoms suggesting a gynaecological problem, such as worsening of symptoms with their periods, pelvic pain (area 8 in Figure 4 on page 49) or pain on intercourse. Obviously, it is very important to make sure that a gynaecological problem is not being missed but there is a tendency for doctors to over-diagnose gynaecological conditions in IBS. This can lead to unnecessary treatment which doesn't help because there wasn't a gynaecological problem in the first place. This tends to happen most if an ultrasound scan reveals an ovarian cyst. If it is small it is unlikely to be causing pain and might be better left alone. However, it is important that ovarian cancer is not missed and a blood test called a CA125 in conjunction with a scan can usually answer this question. This test can even be used as a screening test for ovarian cancer.

Another condition that can cause a lot of confusion is endometriosis. This is a very common condition where pieces of the lining on the womb (the endometrium) can be found outside the womb, either in the ovaries or in other parts of the abdomen. The only way to definitely diagnose this condition is by passing a camera into the abdomen via the tummy button (umbilicus) and this is called a laparoscopy. If it is detected but very mild, it should probably be left alone as treating endometriosis when the pain is due to IBS rather than endometriosis can actually make the pain worse. When the endometriosis is more severe, then it needs treatment from the gynaecologist. However, if there is any doubt, then it is probably safer to treat the person for IBS first and if there is no progress, then reconsider the possibility that the endometriosis is causing the pain.

## What to expect when you go to see your doctor about symptoms that could be due to IBS

If you are under the age of 50 with the typical symptoms described above, the diagnosis of IBS is almost certain especially if you also have some non-colonic symptoms (see page 58).

Your doctor will ask you questions that might make them want to check that nothing else is going on (so called 'red flags'). These include:

- Whether you have had any weight loss.
- If you have any rectal bleeding, especially if it is not associated with anal pain or soreness.
- Whether you have a family history of coeliac disease, Crohn's disease, ulcerative colitis, bowel cancer or ovarian cancer.

They will also want to examine your tummy which may be tender but there should be no lumps or bumps. They may also need to do a rectal examination, especially if you have had some bleeding.

If there are no red flags and examination is normal, they will do a couple of tests just to be on the safe side. These include:

- A blood count to make sure you are not anaemic, which is when your haemoglobin level is low. This is usually due to you being deficient in iron because you are losing it (for example, with heavy periods), because you are not absorbing it (for example, coeliac disease) or because there is not enough iron in your diet. Irritable bowel syndrome does not cause anaemia and, therefore, the cause needs to be investigated and identified.

- A blood test for inflammatory markers (CRP and white blood cell count). The commonest gut-related cause for inflammation is Crohn's disease or ulcerative colitis.

- A blood test for coeliac disease. It is advisable for all people with IBS to have a test for coeliac disease. This is because the symptoms of coeliac disease can be similar to IBS and will be improved by a gluten-free diet. There are two possible tests but it is only necessary to do one as they are equally accurate. The first one looks for endomysial antibodies (EMA) and the second is called the tissue transglutaminase test (tTG).

- If you have diarrhoea, your doctor may want to do a faecal calprotectin test (on your stools) which is a test for inflammation in the bowel (Crohn's disease or ulcerative colitis) which, if negative, saves you having to have a colonoscopy. If it is positive you would have to have a colonoscopy to confirm that you do have inflammation in the gut.

- If you are over 50 it would probably be advisable to have a colonoscopy, especially if you have a family history of bowel cancer. However, one way of screening for bowel cancer is to have your doctor check your stools for traces of blood (faecal occult blood test, see page 57). If it is positive, a colonoscopy would be necessary. However, it is important to remember that there are many causes for traces of blood in the stools, such as a sore bottom, so it doesn't necessarily mean that you have bowel cancer.

Once all this is done, we can get onto the next chapters where you can learn how your IBS can be treated and brought under control, firstly with diet (Chapter 5) and then with other approaches (Chapters 6–8).

# TREATMENT – DIETARY MANIPULATION

When treating IBS it is really important that you try one approach (diet or medication) at a time because, if you try several at once and benefit, you won't know which treatment has helped.

Most people with IBS say that eating makes their symptoms worse. Therefore, it is not surprising that they think they have a dietary allergy or intolerance and usually ask if they can have a diet sheet.

Dietary allergy, where you get an instant reaction to food, is actually quite unusual in IBS. It is more likely to be a problem in people with either eczema, asthma or hay fever and is often easier to recognise because of the immediate nature of the reaction. If a dietary allergy is suspected, there are tests that can be done to identify the cause. In contrast, dietary intolerances are extremely common in IBS and a lot can be done to relieve symptoms by manipulating the diet. Even in people without IBS, certain foods are more 'irritant' to the gut than others and it is, therefore, not surprising that these foods tend to irritate IBS. Unfortunately, the more irritant foods tend to be the ones that are regarded as 'healthy'. Therefore, it is sometimes necessary to find a balance between not eating too healthily and not eating too unhealthily.

## Fibre

It is recommended that we all eat a high-fibre diet as it is thought that such a diet keeps us in good health and reduces the chance of getting bowel cancer or heart disease. There is evidence to suggest that eating a high-fibre diet has a beneficial effect on the fats in the blood but the evidence is not quite so strong with regard to reducing bowel cancer. Fibre does encourage the growth of good bacteria and appears to increase the diversity of the bacteria in the gut microbiome which is considered to be a good thing.

A whole range of complex carbohydrates (carbohydrates joined together in long chains, making them less soluble) can be considered as dietary fibre which is very confusing for the consumer who just wants a simple message. Traditionally, fibre is divided into soluble and insoluble fibre, but some people are not happy with this definition and suggest it should be abandoned because it is not entirely accurate in terms of the 'solubility' of fibre. They suggest that fibre should be defined as 'the edible part of a plant that is resistant to digestion and absorption by the small bowel' but that doesn't help people with IBS make decisions about how their diet might be affecting their symptoms.

However, dividing fibre into soluble and insoluble fibre is helpful because they have differing effects on the gut, which is obviously important to know. Consequently, for the purposes of this book, we are going to stick to the terms soluble and insoluble as they are so much more useful from a practical point of view with respect to treatment. The best examples of insoluble fibre are the breakfast cereals that contain the whole grain, with bran products containing the most. Soluble fibre is found in certain fruit and vegetables and is available commercially in the form of derivatives of ispaghula (psyllium) such as Fybogel or Metamucil. Table 6 lists some of the foods that contain either soluble or insoluble fibre.

---

**Table 6** Some examples of foods that contain soluble or insoluble fibre

**Soluble fibre**

- Oats
- Root vegetables
- Fruit
- Psyllium/ispaghula

**Insoluble fibre**

- Brown bread
- Wholemeal bread
- Wholegrain breakfast cereals
- Digestive biscuits
- Crispbreads
- Some cereal bars
- Seeds

---

A high-fibre diet has, for many years, been recommended as the first-line treatment option for people with IBS. However, fibre tends to have a laxative action as a result of 'irritating' the gut and is, therefore, more likely to irritate an irritable bowel. We have shown that insoluble fibre in the form of bran makes far more people with IBS worse than it makes better (see Table 7).

**Table 7** Percentage of patients with IBS being made better or worse by a variety of different food products

| Fibre source | Better | Worse | Unchanged |
| --- | --- | --- | --- |
| Bran | 11% | 55% | 35% |
| Cornflakes | 0% | 0% | 100% |
| Rice Krispies | 0% | 0% | 100% |
| Porridge | 0% | 12% | 88% |
| Muesli | 0% | 27% | 73% |
| Vegetables | 3% | 25% | 72% |
| Fruit | 5% | 45% | 50% |
| Pulses | 0% | 25% | 75% |
| Nuts | 0% | 27% | 73% |
| Proprietary fibre | 39% | 22% | 39% |

Adapted from *The Lancet* 1994; 344:39–40

Soluble fibre, such as psyllium/ispaghula, does improve symptoms in some people, but can still cause problems in others. Fibre can sometimes improve constipation but, in the case of the insoluble variety, at the expense of causing more bloating, pain and gas. Consequently if you do want to try fibre for your constipation, you should probably only use soluble fibre and we prefer the psyllium/ispaghula derivatives. If you have a tendency to diarrhoea, then you should be wary of all forms of fibre.

Most people are on a fairly high-fibre diet by the time they come to us, so we recommend they cut out the foods listed in Table 8 (overleaf) for a month to see what happens and suggest you might want to try the same, if you have not done this before. If there is an improvement in your symptoms then you know that you have a degree of intolerance to some or all of this type of food product. You can then slowly reintroduce them, one at a time, to try and work out which ones cause the most problems. In some people it is only one or two, in others it may be more – everybody will be different in what they can tolerate. If you are constipated and this gets worse with this change in your diet, but you feel better in other ways, you may need to take a laxative (see page 81). It is sometimes preferable to take a laxative to improve bowel function than to use fibre. It is surprising how many people derive some benefit from this simple change in their diet, but of course, it doesn't work for everyone and you should definitely not carry on with it if you get worse. If you don't improve, you may then want to try the FODMAP diet which is described next.

**Table 8** Reduced-fibre diet

## Foods you can eat

- White bread
- White pasta
- White rice
- Anything made with white flour, e.g. biscuits like Rich Tea, cakes, white sauces
- Rice Krispies – these have added vitamins so you don't need supplements
- Cream crackers

## Foods to avoid

- Brown bread, including wholemeal or granary bread or bread with seeds
- Brown pasta
- Brown rice
- Anything made with wholemeal or brown flour
- All breakfast cereals except Rice Krispies
- Bran
- Digestive biscuits
- Crispbreads
- Cereal bars
- Maize, e.g. cornflakes, tortilla chips, sweetcorn
- Rye, e.g. rye bread, crispbreads
- Oats, e.g. porridge, flapjacks
- Nuts

## Fruit and vegetables

As can be seen from Table 7 as page 66, our study showed that fruit and vegetables can cause problems but, at the time, we were not entirely sure why this should be, as not all fruit and vegetables contain a lot of fibre. This question has recently been answered by the discovery that IBS can be upset by fermentable carbohydrates known as FODMAPs (fermentable oligo-, di- and monosaccharides and polyols), which are found in a variety of different fruit and vegetables. This has led to the introduction of the FODMAP diet which involves excluding those foods which have high amounts of FODMAPs. Some examples of high and low FODMAP foods are listed in Table 9.

**Table 9** Examples of foods high and low in FODMAPs

| High | Low |
| --- | --- |
| Bread | Gluten-free bread |
| Apple | Banana |
| Pear | Blueberry |
| Plum | Rhubarb |
| Watermelon | Lemon |
| Blackberry | Mandarin |
| Peach | Potato |
| Prune | Carrot |
| Cauliflower | Swede |

| High | Low |
|------|-----|
| Sweetcorn | Parsnip |
| Onion | Turnip |
| Garlic | Sugar |
| Leek | All meat |
| Mushroom | All fish |
| Honey | Egg |
| Artificial sweeteners | Rice |
| Cows' milk | Water |

Consequently, if removing cereal fibre doesn't help the situation, it is then worth trying a low FODMAP diet for a period of about four weeks, in addition to your low-fibre diet. There are some good apps available on the internet, especially those from Monash University in Australia and King's College London, and it would also be a good idea to let your general practitioner know that you are doing the diet so they can advise you if necessary.

If the low FODMAP diet leads to an improvement in your symptoms, you will then have to try a slow reintroduction of the items you left out, one by one, to try and work out which ones cause problems. Remember, some will cause more problems than others but if you eat enough of even the relatively trouble-free foods, the FODMAP content could add up to the extent that they could still upset you. In other words, fruit and vegetables will all have a particular 'dose' effect on you and you have to work out what dose your particular gastrointestinal system can tolerate.

Just to complicate things further, in addition to FODMAPs, fruit and vegetables also contain fibre. It may not be quite as irritating to the gut as cereal fibre but it may still cause problems in some people. Therefore, you may have to be wary of some of the more fibrous fruit and vegetables such as oranges, cabbage, broccoli, tomatoes and potato skins. Nuts can also be a problem. Fruit and vegetables can be a particular problem in people with the diarrhoea version of IBS. Carrots are very well tolerated and the inside of a potato hardly upsets anybody with IBS, but the skin of a baked potato can be big trouble!

## Fats and proteins

People with IBS tend to be intolerant of any type of fatty food and often feel better if they avoid consuming excessive amounts of fat. Consequently, semi-skimmed is preferable to full-fat milk and it is better to stick to leaner cuts of meat. If your pain is in the right hypochondrium (area 1 in Figure 4 on page 49), then fat intolerance can raise the suspicion of gallstones and it is important you don't have surgery unless there is a firm diagnosis of gall bladder disease (see page 50).

Fortunately, protein hardly ever upsets people with IBS, although some say that red meat isn't quite so easily digested. Eggs are usually reasonably well tolerated. Most people, even those without IBS, will have a food which tends to not entirely suit them. Therefore, if you are upset by a food that is not usually a problem in IBS, it is best avoided as you are clearly intolerant of it for some reason.

## Gluten and wheat sensitivity

Coeliac disease is a condition where gluten, which is found in wheat and some other cereals (such as rye, barley and oats), damages the lining of the small bowel. The treatment is complete gluten exclusion for life and, in the majority of sufferers, their symptoms, which can be rather similar to IBS, improve considerably. However, in some people with coeliac disease, the IBS symptoms can continue and these should be treated in exactly the same way as IBS, especially if these people are strictly following their gluten-free diet.

Some people with IBS appear to be genuinely sensitive to gluten, although the screening blood test for coeliac disease is negative, as well as the biopsy (tissue sample) taken from the lining of the small bowel. This condition is called non-coeliac gluten sensitivity and in these individuals wheat doesn't appear to be damaging the gut in any way, but they should be advised to continue avoiding gluten if doing this seems to be improving their symptoms. If you suspect you are gluten intolerant, despite having negative tests for coeliac disease, it is perfectly reasonable to exclude gluten entirely from your diet for a month or two to see if it leads to an improvement. If it does, you can continue with gluten exclusion and, if it doesn't, at least you know that gluten does not seem to be a problem in your particular case. An important thing to remember is that in coeliac disease, gluten is damaging the gut and should be left out indefinitely even if it doesn't help your symptoms, whereas in gluten intolerance the consumption of gluten will make symptoms worse, but it will not actually damage the gut in any way. As we have already seen the FODMAP diet excludes gluten as well as other foods from the diet. However, if you just want to test specifically for gluten intolerance, it is perfectly reasonable to exclude gluten on its own for a month or two to see if you experience any beneficial effects.

In other IBS sufferers wheat seems to be the problem rather than any other gluten-containing foods. If you want to try a wheat-free diet it is important to remember that wheat can occur in a whole variety of products, such as some gravy powders, so it is important to read the labels carefully.

## Lactose malabsorption

Lactose is a carbohydrate that occurs in milk and in most people it is digested reasonably well by the gastrointestinal system without any problem. However, in some people the gut doesn't make enough lactase, which is the enzyme that breaks down lactose (see Table 1 on page 6). This results in lactose not being absorbed and, consequently, it is fermented by bacteria in the gut, leading to symptoms. If such a person also has IBS then lactose can cause even more problems. Lactose malabsorption varies considerably depending on race and is relatively common in Asians but much less common in Caucasians. It can also run in families. Lactose malabsorption is easily diagnosed by the use of a breath test which can be done in most hospitals. If you do find out that you have lactose malabsorption, you should moderate your consumption of milk products or even consider using lactose-free milk, although this is more expensive than ordinary milk. Many people find that it is sufficient to just reduce their lactose intake rather than eliminating it from their diet altogether. Lactose is frequently used as a 'filler' in various tablets but, fortunately, not many people have to take lactose exclusion to the extent of also being wary of lactose in tablets. Just as with other intolerances, lactose will not damage your bowel if you do consume it but, obviously, doing so will probably make your symptoms worse.

The other constituents of milk that can sometimes cause symptoms are fat and protein. Fat as a cause of problems with milk can be relatively easily ruled out by just drinking skimmed milk. If skimmed milk still upsets you and you don't have lactose intolerance, you may have milk protein intolerance, although this is quite unusual. There are several different proteins in milk, although casein is the most abundant and there are two main types of casein which vary according to source. For instance, some breeds of cow have more of one type than others and this may explain why some people find they can better tolerate a particular type of milk. If you do decide to try excluding milk from your diet for a while, it is important to remember milk products are contained in a wide range of foods. If you do have milk protein intolerance or just don't like milk, probably the best substitute is rice milk. Many people use either soya milk or almond milk but these two substitutes are not always well tolerated by IBS sufferers.

## Sugar substitutes

The consumption of sugar substitutes such as sorbitol and fructose has increased enormously over recent years and they are now widely used by the food industry. Unfortunately, most of these substances are fermentable carbohydrates (FODMAPs) and, therefore, can upset IBS. Consequently, you need to be cautious about the consumption of sugar-free drinks and diet products that may contain these particular sweeteners. Aspartame is often used instead of sugar and does not seem to cause as many problems although some people with IBS find that even this product can appear to upset their symptoms. Interestingly, ordinary sugar seldom upsets IBS symptoms although it is obviously a source of excess calories.

## Tests for dietary intolerances

The screening test for coeliac disease (see page 55) is very reliable and tests for true dietary allergy are relatively straightforward and are available on the NHS. However, dietary allergy is unusual in IBS and there are no reliable tests for intolerances. Testing the blood for antibodies to food (IgG antibodies) is very controversial, although there is one study suggesting it may be useful in some individuals, but it is very expensive. Other tests for dietary intolerance have not been shown to be of any use in IBS and are, therefore, probably best avoided.

## Food diaries

It is often suggested that a food diary can help with working out which foods are causing trouble. We don't find this approach very useful because when you have an intolerance to a certain food, the effect may take a few days to come on. In addition the 'dose' of that food may be important. For instance, if you eat a food to which you have some degree of intolerance once a week it may not affect you, but if you have it every day it may cause problems.

## Wind

Gas and wind have been discussed elsewhere (see page 16) but it is important to remember that what you eat can make you more windy and this applies particularly to the high-fibre foods. Wind is even more troublesome when it smells badly. This problem can often be improved by being careful about your intake of particular foods, although different people find different foods make their wind more smelly. Consequently, you have to work out which foods affect you most. Some of the most troublesome foods with regard to causing a bad smell include broccoli, cabbage, sprouts, cauliflower, onions, eggs and sometimes red meat such as beef. Like everything to do with diet, 'dose' is important so go easy with the foods that you know cause problems especially when in company.

## How to manage all this dietary information

Making big changes to your diet, as has been mentioned here, can be quite challenging for an IBS sufferer, especially as some of the advice is almost the opposite of what we are given today in order to try and stay healthy. Fortunately, our patients have a helpline they can call, but if your IBS is significantly upsetting your life, it is still worth trying a change in your diet even without the luxury of a helpline. Obviously, if your IBS is very mild, you should just be reading this as an educational exercise rather than necessarily changing your diet. It is always useful to know about those foods that can potentially upset IBS as opposed to those that don't usually cause problems.

It is a pity that the internet is rather confusing about diet and IBS, with often conflicting advice or even misinformation about which foods are good for the condition. Don't forget that every individual person is different, therefore, what suits one person may not suit another. Unfortunately, 'healthy' foods have a tendency to sometimes irritate IBS which is confusing for the sufferer who wants to try and eat as healthily as possible but at the same time minimise their symptoms. Most people can find a happy medium between these two extremes by a process of trial and error and find it easier to cope once they have a good idea of which foods seem to cause the most problems.

It is really useful to know your 'safe' and 'unsafe' foods, although there may be some foods that you can't be sure about. Consequently, when you are going through a bad patch, you can restrict yourself to just your 'safe' foods until things settle down again. Even if one of your favourite foods seems to make your symptoms worse, you may occasionally want to 'let yourself go' because, if you suffer the consequences, at least you know why and you also know it is not actually harming you in any way. The important thing to remember is that you are gradually taking control and your symptoms are becoming predictable, rather than unpredictable, which is what people with IBS find so frustrating.

# CHAPTER 6

# TREATMENT – MEDICATION AND OTHER APPROACHES

There are a variety of medications available for IBS; some are available over the counter but others need a prescription. Most drugs have two names and some may have even more. A generic name is the actual name of the drug and the brand name, spelled with a capital letter, is the name given to it by the manufacturer. In this chapter we will always refer to the generic name but may give the brand name in brackets if it is particularly well known.

## Antispasmodics

As their name implies, antispasmodics are designed to relieve any spasm in the muscle of the bowel and, therefore, the pain. There are two main types of antispasmodic medication: one is called a smooth muscle relaxant and the other an anticholinergic. The smooth muscle relaxant has a direct relaxing effect on the gut muscle whereas an anticholinergic blocks the nerves that make the muscle contract. Some of these drugs have additional activity, such as analgesic effects, or some have a mixture of smooth muscle relaxing and anticholinergic effects (mixed activity). Table 10 lists some of the various antispasmodics that are available and it is important to note that different antispasmodics are available in different countries.

---

**Table 10** Antispasmodic medications

**Anticholinergics**

- Dicycloverine*
- Hyoscine*
- Otilonium
- Cimetropium
- Dicyclomine
- Trimebutine**
- Pirenzepine
- Rociverine (mixed activity)
- Prifinium
- Propinox (mixed activity)

**Smooth muscle relaxants**

- Mebeverine*
- Alverine*
- Pinaverium

*readily available in the UK
**also has additional analgesic activity

---

People with IBS vary in their response to different antispasmodics and it is sometimes worth trying several and choosing the one that suits you best. There is little to be gained in taking more than one of the same type but you can combine an anticholinergic with a smooth muscle relaxant. One particular antispasmodic called hyoscine butylbromide (Buscopan) is not very well absorbed from the gut so it is sometimes worth taking a slightly higher dose (four tablets instead of two) to see if you can get a better effect. Antispasmodics are extremely safe, have very few side-effects and can be taken on an indefinite basis if necessary. The smooth muscle relaxants can occasionally cause mild constipation and the anticholinergics can also have this effect, as well as sometimes giving a dry mouth. The majority of these medications are available over the counter and can be used regularly or 'as necessary', according to whether your IBS is intermittent or continuous.

## Laxatives

The laxatives commonly used in the UK are listed in Table 11 (overleaf). Some stimulate the bowel (stimulant laxatives) and some 'suck' water into the bowel from the bloodstream (osmotic laxatives) or soften the stool (softeners). If you are only intermittently constipated, it is reasonable to just take a laxative when you need one. However, if your bowels are sluggish most of the time, it is far better to take a laxative every day in order to try and mimic, as much as possible, a normal bowel habit. Consequently, you should take a small dose of a laxative all the time rather than a large dose intermittently, which will often lead to a much more unpredictable response. People vary considerably in their response to laxatives so each person has to find the dose that suits them, which can be completely different to someone else who has a similar degree of constipation.

**Table 11** Commonly used laxatives

| | |
|---|---|
| **Osmotic** | Polyethylene glycol (macrogol, Movicol, Laxido) |
| | Lactulose |
| | Magnesium salts |
| **Stimulant** | Bisacodyl |
| | Senna |
| | Sodium picosulfate |
| **Softeners** | Docusate |

Laxatives are usually best taken last thing at night but the lag time between taking the medication and getting an effect varies from person to person, so some people have to take them at a different time. You should aim to take a dose at a time that gives a predictable response, which is under control and doesn't interfere with your day-to-day activities. Most people feel much better for having a good 'clear out' every day as constipation can lead to headaches, bad breath, an unpleasant taste in the mouth and feeling very sluggish. It is a complete fallacy that laxatives damage the bowel and, if necessary, you can take laxatives indefinitely without any fear of them causing long-term problems. The most commonly used laxative in the UK is macrogol (Movicol or Laxido). If you are constipated, your bowel is already a bit lazy so taking a laxative will definitely not make it lazier. It is perfectly acceptable to take other IBS medications, such as an antispasmodic, with a laxative.

## Antidiarrhoeals

The most commonly used medication for diarrhoea is loper-amide (Imodium) which is very effective and extremely safe. Rather like with laxatives, people vary in the dose required to get a satisfactory response and this medication can be taken regularly or 'as necessary'. It can even be used pre-emptively (as a precaution) if you are having to do something where you do not want to be 'let down' by your bowels.

Loperamide has virtually no side-effects but, not surpris-ingly, can lead to constipation if you don't get the dose right. However, the constipation will rapidly clear if you reduce the dose or stop it for a while. Loperamide does not usually relieve pain and, in some people, can occasionally lead to more dis-comfort or bloating. As loperamide does not help pain, it is perfectly reasonable to take an antispasmodic for the pain as well as loperamide to control the bowel habit. Some people will become constipated after taking even one capsule of lop-eramide, which at least shows the drug works for them. In this situation it is worth pulling the capsule apart and taking a half or a quarter of the contents to see if you can find a dose that suits you. Other people may need to take as many as eight or ten capsules in a day to get control. The duration of the effect of loperamide varies from person to person and, therefore, each individual has to work out how long it works for them and adjust the timing of consumption accordingly.

Loperamide is often used for gastroenteritis but it is important to remember that in this situation the diarrhoea is serving a purpose by 'flushing' out the cause of the infection. Consequently, it is important not to constipate yourself with loperamide when you have a gastrointestinal infection. In addition, if you have colitis (ulcerative colitis or Crohn's disease, see page 44) it is important to avoid loperamide during attacks, as this can lead to a build-up of fluid in the bowel which may cause serious problems. Fortunately, in IBS the diarrhoea is serving no useful purpose and can be suppressed without any fear of damaging your bowel.

Ondansetron (Zofran) is a medication that was introduced many years ago for the treatment of nausea and vomiting associated with chemotherapy. It is a remarkably safe drug but does tend to cause constipation. This makes it potentially useful for the treatment of diarrhoea-type IBS and studies have confirmed that it does have a beneficial effect, especially on urgency. Unfortunately, it doesn't seem to help pain very much but, because of its 'anti-nausea' action, it can help nausea which is a very common symptom in IBS. Although not as common as nausea, vomiting can be a problem in some people with IBS and ondansetron can also help to relieve this symptom. Ondansetron is only available on prescription.

Codeine is sometimes used to relieve diarrhoea and, because it is also a painkiller related to morphine, it can help with pain control. However, it is very addictive if taken on a regular basis and, therefore, we strongly discourage its continuous use. It is bad enough having IBS – we don't want to add 'drug dependency' to the problem!

Diphenoxylate and atropine (Lomotil) is another diarrhoea medication that is available over the counter. It is also called co-phenotrope. Like codeine, it is also related to morphine so, again, is probably best avoided unless nothing else helps.

# Probiotics

A probiotic is an organism, usually a bacteria, which is good for you. As we have already seen on page 18, our bowel contains many bacteria that actually keep us in good health by, for example, boosting our immune system. There is evidence that people with IBS have dysbiosis which is the name given to an abnormal microbiome (see page 118). There seems to be a deficiency of good bacteria in some people with IBS and, therefore, it seems reasonable to give probiotics to try and put this right. Probiotics have a wide range of potentially useful activities and these are listed in Table 12.

---

**Table 12** Some of the properties of probiotics

- Boost the immune response
- Help to reduce inflammation
- Improve the ability of the gut to stop germs crossing it and getting into the body.
- Inhibit the growth of dangerous (pathogenic) bacteria
- Reduce the ability of viruses to attach to cells
- Make chemicals that can kill bacteria
- Make chemicals that can inactivate toxins made by bacteria
- Appear to influence the function of our central nervous system

---

A particular probiotic may have one or more of these properties, but it is unlikely that there is a probiotic that has all of them.

The majority of probiotics that have been tried in IBS belong to either the lactobacillae or bifidobacteria families. The important thing to remember is that all probiotic organisms are different from each other unless they have exactly the same name. For example, if 'lactobacillus type A' can improve the symptoms of IBS, it doesn't mean that 'lactobacillus type B' will also be effective. The good thing about probiotics is that they are harmless and do not seem to cause any side-effects. They are most commonly available in capsule form or yoghurts. Probiotics are not available on prescription for IBS but are widely available in pharmacies, health food shops and supermarkets.

The problem is that not many probiotics have been studied and been shown to help the symptoms of IBS. That doesn't mean to say they don't help, it just means that they haven't been tested for that purpose. We have tested a couple of probiotics (bifidobacterium infantis 35624 and lactobacillus lactis CNCM 1-2494) and found them to be helpful. The best approach to taking a probiotic is to try one for a month or two and, if it helps, continue with it, probably on a long-term basis.

Don't expect a probiotic to have a dramatic effect on your symptoms like taking a paracetamol for a headache, where you will know within hours whether it is effective or not. Probiotics should be seen as slow-acting preparations that will gradually lead to a more general improvement in your condition rather than necessarily relieving one particular symptom. Remember, that just because a yoghurt is called a bioyoghurt, it may not contain sufficient bacteria to have an effect and, of course, some people do not like yoghurts or can't tolerate dairy products. Hopefully, in the future, 'designer' probiotics will become available which are specifically made for use in IBS.

## Prebiotics

A prebiotic is a product that encourages the growth of your own 'good bacteria'. There has not been much research on their effect in IBS although one study has suggested that a trans-galactooligosaccharide (GOS) appears to be beneficial in some patients. This result is somewhat confusing because GOS is a FODMAP and, as we have already seen, FODMAPs can cause problems in IBS (see page 69). This suggests that some FODMAPs may be less 'harmful' to the gut than others or may even be beneficial. Some companies are now marketing probiotics with an added prebiotic to 'boost' the effect of the probiotic. This combination of prebiotic and probiotic is called a synbiotic or symbiotic and it may be that these preparations may also help IBS.

## Antidepressants

As we have seen on pages 17 and 43, there is a strong connection between the gut and the brain (gut–brain axis) and many of the chemicals in the brain responsible for its activity (neurotransmitters) are also found in the gut. It is, therefore, not surprising to find that drugs, such as antidepressants, which can affect the activity of the brain, may also have an effect on the gut.

**Table 13** Antidepressants that are used in IBS

**Tricyclic antidepressants**

- Amitryptiline
- Nortriptyline
- Imipramine
- Clomipramine
- Desipramine
- Trimipramine
- Doxepin
- Dosulepin

**Selective serotonin re-uptake inhibitors**

- Fluoxetine
- Paroxetine
- Citalopram
- Escitalopram
- Fluvoxamine
- Sertraline

**Others**

- Duloxetine
- Mirtazapine

There are several 'classes' of antidepressants but the two that are most commonly used in IBS are the tricyclic anti-depressants (TCAs) and the selective serotonin re-uptake inhibitors (SSRIs). Table 13 lists these drugs, of which ami-triptyline (Tryptizol) and fluoxetine (Prozac) are two of the more well-known examples. Amitriptyline is the TCA that is most frequently used in IBS and can be very effective in relieving many of the symptoms, especially the abdominal pain. Fortunately, it works at about a tenth of the dose required for depression and, therefore, the side-effects are not as troublesome when used to treat IBS compared to depression. That does mean that if you also want a TCA to improve a low mood, this is unlikely to happen because the dose will not be high enough to have a beneficial effect on mood. However, if a low mood is the result of the IBS, then a TCA may help as a result of improving the IBS rather than having a direct effect on mood. TCAs have been shown to reduce gastrointestinal hypersensitivity suggesting that this might be one way by which they improve IBS symptoms. The main side-effect of amitriptyline is sleepiness but that can be managed reasonably well by starting at a very low dose and taking the medication at night. If the dose needs to be increased, then it should all be taken at night. This drug also tends to constipate slightly so that means it is especially effective in the diarrhoea variety of IBS. It can also be used in constipation-type IBS, but a laxative may also be needed or, if you are already taking a laxative, the dose may need increasing. Dry mouth can also be a bit of a problem and, like any drug, some people just can't tolerate amitriptyline at all. The side-effects tend to wear off after a week or two so it is worth persevering, but it does not suit everyone. We find that about 60–70 per cent of people derive worthwhile benefits from amitriptyline but it does usually have to be taken on a long-term basis. TCAs are not addictive but, if you decide to stop them, it is best to tail them off slowly.

SSRIs can be tried, especially if a TCA has not proved effective or you have not been able to tolerate it for some reason. SSRIs have to be used at the same dose used for depression and have different side-effects to the TCAs. These include loose bowels, which can be an advantage in a constipated person, and nausea, which usually wears off after a week or two. We do not find them quite as effective as TCAs for IBS but they can be very useful if you also have a very low mood. We usually use citalopram as this is the mildest SSRI with the lowest rate of side-effects and probably causes the least dependency. However, if you happen to be on a different SSRI, it would not be worth changing to citalopram, as there is very little to choose between them other than dependency, which tends to be a little higher with the others. If you can't tolerate a TCA or an SSRI, then mirtazapine or duloxetine are worth considering.

Many people with IBS are reluctant to take an antidepressant as they think we are just using these drugs because we think they are depressed. However, if you remember that the brain and the gut are closely connected and are made up of similar nerves that use similar chemical transmitters, then it comes as no surprise that drugs that work on the brain are likely to have similar effects on the gut. It is best to just try them for a few months and, if they don't have any beneficial effects, they can always be stopped.

## Simethicone

Wind in either direction, up or down, can be a major problem in IBS and, as we have already seen, diet can be helpful in bringing this under control. Unfortunately, there are no really effective medications for this problem, although simethicone can sometimes prove to be helpful. It is contained in a number of over the counter preparations from pharmacies and it is always worth trying one or more of these to see if they prove helpful.

## New drugs

Until recently, we have not had a new IBS drug in the UK for over 20 years. This is partly because the regulatory authorities have not taken IBS very seriously in the past and have, therefore, demanded absolute safety from any new medication. This is clearly unattainable as it is impossible to develop a drug that has no side-effects at all. However, the climate is changing a little and the pharmaceutical industry is now taking more of an interest in IBS. As a consequence, some new drugs are appearing and more are in the pipeline. Many of the current medications for IBS, such as antispasmodics or antidepressants, can be used for any type of IBS, such as people with diarrhoea, constipation or an alternating bowel habit. This is not the case with some of the new drugs which, because of the way they work, are usually targeted at one particular bowel habit abnormality.

So far, we have prucalopride, linaclotide and lubiprostone for constipation and eluxadoline for diarrhoea. They are all prescription medications and currently their availability varies across the UK and even from county to county. At present, it is recommended that they should be used only when the standard medications have been ineffective and, with the constipation medications, some people will respond better to one than another. So, just like with all other approaches to IBS, it is a case of trying one and seeing if it suits you and, if it doesn't, trying another. With the way they are prescribed currently there is little room for adjusting the dose. Hopefully that will change with time as it is likely that some individuals will need different doses depending on the severity of their symptoms.

Rifaximin is an antibiotic which is not absorbed from the gut, so is potentially much safer than other antibiotics. It has been suggested that, as some people with IBS appear to have dysbiosis (see page 118), such an antibiotic might be beneficial in this condition. Trials of rifaximin taken for approximately two weeks in people with IBS suggest an improvement in symptoms in those without constipation and it has been approved for use in this type of IBS in the USA. We will have to see how long symptom improvement lasts after a two-week course of treatment and whether repeated courses bring about the same degree of improvement. Irritable bowel syndrome should be regarded as a lifelong condition, even if the severity fluctuates and, therefore, some people are concerned about the safety of rifaximin if it has to be used over many years.

## Suppositories, enemas and irrigation

Suppositories are torpedo-shaped medications (see Figure 5) designed to be introduced into the rectum where the active ingredient can be released. A whole variety of drugs can be delivered in this way, especially if someone is vomiting or can't swallow medication for any reason. In IBS the most common use of a suppository is to try and stimulate the bowels to open in someone with constipation. The two most frequently used suppositories are glycerin and bisaco-dyl. People vary in their willingness to use this approach to administer a medication but they can be effective, especially if there is not too much of a backlog of stool. There is no evidence that the use of suppositories can be harmful.

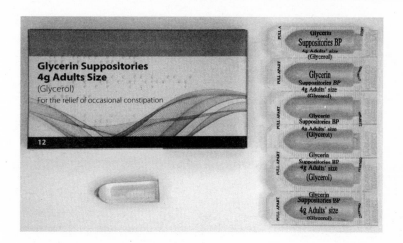

Figure 5 An example of a suppository

An enema is the name given to the process of running fluid into the rectum with the aim of stimulating the bowel and washing it out. In the past, people used to make up their own enema and introduce the liquid, such as soapy water, using a pump or bag on a stand rather like that used to give a person an intravenous drip in hospital. There is a remote chance that this type of enema can damage the bowel, and these days ready-made enemas are available for the treatment of constipation that are much easier and safer to use. The volume of fluid in these ready-made enemas varies from 5 millilitres (Figure 6) to 100 millilitres (Figure 7). Their use is safe in fit and healthy people but, especially with the higher volume versions, the contents can be partially absorbed into the body and cause problems. Consequently, they should be used with caution in people with heart or kidney trouble. It is best to use enemas only with the advice of a doctor.

Many people with IBS say they feel better after colonic irrigation but we are very reluctant to recommend this

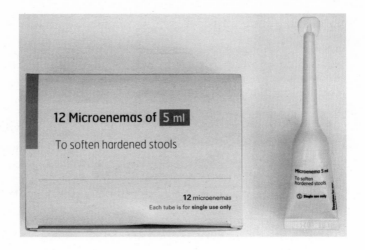

Figure 6 An example of a small volume enema
(microenema) containing 5 ml of fluid

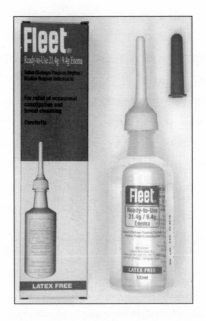

Figure 7 130 ml phosphate (Fleet) enema

approach as ideally this should be done under medical supervision as there is a risk, although small, of perforation of the bowel. However, there is now an alternative, called anal irrigation, that can be offered by the NHS. This comes in the form of a kit that can be used to wash out the last part of the bowel with water and should only be used with the advice of a doctor or a healthcare professional trained in its use. It can be used regularly at home and once you have been instructed how to use it, can be very effective. We use it in people who haven't responded well to laxatives, although sometimes they have to continue using a small dose of a laxative to get the maximum beneficial effect.

## Lifestyle

All the usual healthy lifestyle advice that applies to everybody is equally relevant to people with IBS. Moderate exercise, such as brisk walking, cycling or swimming, depending on personal preference, has been shown to lead to an improvement in symptoms but excessive exercise can actually make the symptoms of IBS worse in some people. There is no doubt that lack of sleep can make IBS worse, but ensuring you get enough sleep can be difficult, especially if your symptoms disrupt your sleep. Eating too late can affect sleep and many IBS sufferers say that they feel better when they eat little and often as opposed to having one large meal at the end of the day. An adequate fluid intake is important but should not be excessive, especially as so many people with IBS have a bit of an 'irritable bladder'. If you are constipated, it is important to avoid dehydration, but taking a lot of fluid does not cure the problem, so it is important to get the balance right.

The sensation of needing to open the bowels is most commonly at its height in the morning and is usually increased by having breakfast (the gastrocolonic response, see page 14) and then disappears for the rest of the day. Some people will ignore this urge to open their bowels, if it is inconvenient, and this is fine as long as they don't do it all the time. However, if you are constipated, it is really important that you use this 'morning urge' to your advantage and ensure you have some breakfast and a hot drink to maximise its effect as much as possible.

With regard to fluid intake, still water is the best choice as fizzy drinks, colas and cordials can cause problems. When alcohol causes a problem it seems to occur more with beers, lagers and wine, whereas gin and vodka seem to be less troublesome. For some reason, tea appears to cause less trouble than coffee, suggesting that caffeine is not the whole problem, although even tea should not be drunk to excess.

There is no doubt that in some people with IBS stopping smoking can make their symptoms worse. In addition, many people with constipation say that a cigarette helps them to open their bowels. However, the detrimental effects of smoking on health are so serious that we cannot recommend that patients with IBS should continue smoking. The one exception to this rule is when we are trying to treat a very severe patient where we sometimes suggest that they should defer stopping smoking until we have been able to get their condition under some degree of control.

## Surgery

As a general rule, surgery has no role in the management of IBS and usually makes symptoms worse. Occasionally, someone with diverticular disease (see page 51) and very serious narrowing of the bowel may need to have the narrow segment removed, but this is very unusual. Some people have constipation that is so severe that they can go for many weeks without opening their bowels, even with massive doses of laxatives. In this situation an operation may be considered but, again, this is extremely unusual.

Haemorrhoids and anal fissures (see page 30) are quite common in IBS and often improve if the IBS can be brought under control. However, sometimes IBS sufferers with these problems are offered surgery. In the case of haemorrhoids this can be something minor like banding, where a rubber band is put round the haemorrhoids to shrink them, or actual removal which is called a haemorrhoidectomy. Although quite painful, banding does not usually cause too much trouble but, as patients with IBS tend to not do well with surgery, we usually advise against haemorrhoidectomy unless there is absolutely no alternative. Similarly, one of the operations for an anal fissure is an anal stretch, although we usually recommend a more conservative treatment such as botox injections, especially in the first instance.

Gynaecological surgery, such as hysterectomy or prolapse repair, may make the symptoms of IBS worse so it is very important that the reason for doing such surgery is very clear. Obviously, if there is a definite gynaecological abnormality there is no question that an operation should be done. However if, for instance, a hysterectomy is being advised in the hope that it might help tummy pain low down in the pelvis, caution is necessary. Similarly, prolapse repair can be extremely helpful but it is important to remember that IBS can be associated with bladder as well as bowel symptoms, so repair of a minor prolapse needs to be considered carefully as the symptoms may actually be due to IBS and not the prolapse.

## Putting it all together

The best way to treat IBS is to go through all the options from diet to medication, one by one, in order to find out what suits a particular person. It is nearly always worth everybody with IBS trying some degree of dietary manipulation but, obviously, some treatments are specific for certain symptoms, such as laxatives for constipation, antidiarrhoeals for diarrhoea and antispasmodics for pain. However, combinations of treatments are often needed so, for instance, if diet helps to some extent it may be that an antispasmodic will be necessary for more severe episodes of pain. If reducing fibre helps but tends to constipate, then adding in a laxative may be a better option than resorting to more fibre. If your IBS does not respond well to diet, antispasmodics and laxatives (or antidiarrhoeals), you should not be afraid of trying an antidepressant, as they can be very effective and you can always stop them if they don't work or they cause side-effects. They can be combined with all other IBS medications but should be taken all the time rather than taking them now and again.

In some people one symptom is predominant and they say they can put up with the rest. Consequently, if it is pain then we have to concentrate on trying the antispasmodics, whereas if it is abnormal bowel function laxatives or antidiarrhoeals will be needed. Some symptoms are more difficult to improve than others, with bloating often being particularly resistant to treatment. Reducing fibre, fruit and vegetables probably helps bloating the most although relieving any constipation is also important. Unfortunately the effect of antispasmodics on bloating is often disappointing and its response to antidepressants is patchy, but they are worth trying. Sometimes, someone will say one of their non-colonic symptoms, especially constant lethargy or tiredness, is the main problem. Again, these symptoms are difficult to treat and we find the best way to improve them is to concentrate on improving the IBS in the expectation that the non-colonic symptoms will follow suit.

Some people fail to respond well to any of the measures described in this and the previous chapter and in this situation behavioural treatments need to be considered. These will be covered in the next two chapters.

# CHAPTER 7
# BEHAVIOURAL TREATMENTS

A behavioural therapy is an approach to treatment that involves a therapist helping someone to manage their illness in a variety of ways that do not involve medication. With regard to IBS, the most commonly used techniques are cognitive behavioural therapy (CBT), psychotherapy and hypnotherapy, although mindfulness is now receiving considerable attention. Expressive writing has also been used, although this doesn't necessarily have to involve a therapist. Our Unit has been providing hypnotherapy for IBS for nearly 30 years and, therefore, has huge experience in the use of this form of treatment. Consequently, the next chapter will be devoted entirely to the use of hypnotherapy with the remaining behavioural treatments being described in this chapter.

It is probably not surprising that the possibility of behavioural approaches being helpful in IBS has been investigated, given the importance of the gut–brain axis (see page 17) in this condition. In addition, the fact that antidepressants often improve IBS suggests that targeting the central nervous system (see page 23) is worth considering. Therefore, one way of viewing behavioural approaches is to think of them as a technique for targeting the central nervous system and the enteric nervous system (see page 12) without having to give the drugs that are usually used for this purpose, such as antidepressants. However, it is our opinion that behavioural treatments should not be considered as 'stand alone' treatments and that anything which has a positive effect in IBS, such as diet or medication, should be combined to give the best possible outcome.

There are four potential problems with any behavioural treatment. The first is availability. Not all doctors have access to a particular approach and, therefore, have to use whatever is available. The second issue is the therapist. The relationship between the person with IBS and their therapist is absolutely crucial. Just like in day-to-day life, there are some people who we don't feel quite so comfortable with as others, and that can obviously affect treatment. It is probably fair to say that, if you don't feel comfortable with your therapist, it might be best to try and find someone else, if at all possible. The third problem is that if you do not want to have a particular form of therapy that is being recommended, this will almost certainly reduce its chances of success. However, it might be worth trying it for a couple of sessions, although if you don't like it then it is pointless continuing. The last problem is the content of the therapy. Obviously, there are some basic principles attached to a particular form of therapy, but most therapists will adapt it to their particular style and this may be completely different to the way another therapist gives what is claimed to be exactly the same treatment. There has been very little research on whether one style is better than another or how the content of a session affects the result.

All these problems make it very difficult to give a clear account of what is involved in these various forms of therapy and, therefore, what follows is a general overview of what they entail.

## Cognitive behavioural therapy (CBT)

This form of treatment seeks to change the way an IBS sufferer thinks and behaves in response to their symptoms with the aim of managing them better. Many people with IBS have what is called 'hypervigilance'. This is a medical word for a state where you are checking your body all the time for symptoms. For instance, when you first wake up you may start thinking, 'Have I got any pain?' This makes you concentrate your mind on the area where you usually experience the pain and, even if there is only minimal discomfort, you will then inevitably amplify it and consequently establish a vicious circle. Another feature of IBS is 'catastrophisation'. This is where someone thinks that things are bound to go wrong in a certain situation. For example, if they are asked to go to a function or on a trip, they will immediately start to panic that they may not be able to cope with the situation, even many weeks or months before it is due to happen. Sometimes people find it is easier to just say 'no' and, of course, eventually they don't get asked and become more and more isolated. Some sufferers can even become totally housebound.

Cognitive behavioural therapy aims to try and get people to change these thoughts and, in particular, face their demons. This has to be a slow process of gradually facing a particular issue, often in a graded way. For instance, in a housebound person, it might only be a matter of just going to the front gate initially. In conjunction with these strategies, people are often also given advice on various relaxation techniques and the development of 'safe' thoughts. Cognitive behavioural therapy is usually delivered on a one-to-one basis over a variable length of time, depending on the provider, and has been shown to reduce the symptoms of IBS in a number of different research studies. More recently, CBT programmes designed to be delivered over the internet have been developed and may be useful for those people who are finding it hard to access this form of treatment from their healthcare provider.

## Psychotherapy

Some people with IBS are somewhat reticent about psychotherapy, as the word implies that the problem is 'all in their mind', which, of course, is entirely *un*true. The particular form of psychotherapy that is most often used in IBS is called psychodynamic interpersonal therapy which is sometimes referred to as the conversational model of therapy.

It would be misleading to say that a psychotherapist will not focus on the more psychological aspects of someone's condition and it is obvious that previous events in a person's life will have an impact on how they behave in the future. With regard to IBS, certain events, such as those in relation to previous 'toileting' or 'abuse' experiences, are going to be particularly relevant. Understanding this relationship can then help the sufferer to see why certain symptoms may be more troublesome than others. This form of treatment does not totally concentrate on past psychological issues and also includes techniques used for stress management and relaxation, as well as those used in CBT. There is no doubt that stress can result in IBS becoming more severe but, if someone with IBS is asked whether they had any tummy problems, however mild, before whatever caused the stress, they often say, 'I have always had a funny tummy' or 'My tummy has always been sensitive, especially before something like an exam.' This leads to the idea that the tendency towards IBS has always been present but the stressful event has changed it from a minor nuisance to a major problem. As we have previously seen, IBS sufferers tend to be anxious but only seldom depressed. However, it would be rather surprising if someone with severe tummy pain, bloating and a completely unpredictable bowel habit did not become a bit anxious or down in the dumps as a result of their condition, rather than necessarily being a 'stress head'. Of course, there are some people who are very 'stressy' and that sort of personality will probably suffer more severe symptoms from any illness that they may suffer from, including IBS. Just like all other behavioural treatments, psychotherapy is not suitable for every IBS sufferer and is probably better for those where psychological problems are somewhat more prominent.

## Mindfulness

Mindfulness is a technique that has become very popular in recent years and has been applied to the management of a whole variety of conditions, including IBS. It is the process of concentrating on the present and what is going on around you in terms of thoughts, feelings and your surroundings. This can include what you see, what you hear, as well as what you are thinking, for example, being aware of any sounds going on around you or something like the feel of the chair you are sitting on. People are also encouraged to experience the flow of thoughts going through their mind at the time and, consequently, better understand how some of these can be unhelpful. They are encouraged to accept that thoughts are the result of a normally functioning brain and do not necessarily have to overwhelm us or be taken too seriously. They are encouraged to let thoughts pass without trying to change them, think about them or analyse them. The idea is that this process leads to you becoming less stressed about everything and not ruminating about problems so much.

Mindfulness is also being used to manage a wide variety of situations that we meet on a day-to-day basis, such as issues arising in the workplace. Research is now emerging on the use of mindfulness in a range of medical conditions and there have been some studies in IBS suggesting that it can be helpful in this condition. However, so far, it has not been adopted by the healthcare system in the UK for IBS, so there is the problem of how to access it and knowing whether a particular provider is trustworthy and reliable.

## Expressive writing

It has been shown that if people are encouraged to write about a particular problem that is troubling them in a very frank and honest way, this can help them deal with such issues. Just like some people find it helpful to talk about a problem, some people find it easier to write about it, especially if it is embarrassing. What you have written doesn't necessarily have to be read by somebody else. Some people even find it helpful to destroy or burn what they have written as a way of 'getting rid' of the problem.

All these behavioural techniques have been shown to be of value in the treatment of IBS, although some will appeal more than others to a particular person and, just like all other treatments for IBS, you sometimes have to 'pick and mix' to find the best option for you as an individual.

There have been no comparisons of the various behavioural techniques that have been used to treat IBS. This would be very useful as it might then encourage healthcare services to provide the most effective treatment, if one proved better than the others. Unfortunately, such a comparison is unlikely to happen in the near future because of the problem of the considerable variation in the way these treatments are provided. However, the recent move to record samples of what therapists are doing when they treat people might lead to better consistency in the way these techniques are provided, which would then allow comparisons to be made.

## Biofeedback

Biofeedback is a technique for learning how to try and control a bodily function by connecting the person to an instrument that gives them information about the activity of the particular bodily function that they are attempting to control. For instance, if we wanted someone to learn how to reduce their blood pressure, we could attach them to a device that gives them a visual (for example, a line) or a sound (such as a continuous tone) representation of the current blood pressure. The person is then asked to concentrate their mind on moving the line (for example, down) or changing the pitch of the tone (for example, making it lower) and linking the change in the line or tone to a reduction in their blood pressure. Gradually, with practice, they can learn what thoughts bring about a lowering of their blood pressure, so that eventually they can lower their blood pressure without having to use the device any more.

As we saw on page 30, anismus is one of the causes of constipation where some of the muscles associated with defaecation fail to relax as they should do. We can usually identify this problem relatively easily by placing a small balloon in the rectum and then asking the patient to push it out. If they can't expel the balloon, then they are likely to have anismus and biofeedback can be a solution. Using a device that displays the tension in the muscles that they are not relaxing properly, they can then learn to overcome the problem and start to open their bowels more normally.

There is some evidence that abdominal distension is, at least, partly related to abnormal contraction of the diaphragm (see page 35) and, consequently, biofeedback might also help this problem. Preliminary indications are that it could be helpful, but the only way to get a sensor near the diaphragm is to put it down the oesophagus until it reaches the point where the oesophagus goes through the diaphragm. This is obviously very intrusive and, therefore, it seems unlikely that biofeedback for distension is ever going to be widely available, which is in contrast to its use in anismus which is steadily increasing.

Unfortunately, the availability of the various techniques described in this chapter is rather patchy. Cognitive behavioural therapy is becoming more available on the NHS in the UK and some of the more specialised hospitals can provide biofeedback and psychotherapy. The first person to approach about these other forms of treatment would be your general practitioner and, failing that, it is best to go on recommendation rather than just searching the internet.

# CHAPTER 8
# HYPNOTHERAPY FOR IBS

Unfortunately, hypnosis is a very misunderstood subject, with the activities of stage hypnotists causing even more confusion. This is such a shame as it has great potential in the field of medicine and people need to be reassured that there is no 'loss of control' and you cannot be made to do anything that is 'against your will'. The best way to think about it is as a deep state of relaxation where you can learn to control the various functions of your body through the 'power of your mind'. For instance, with regard to the gastrointestinal system, it has been shown that by using hypnotherapy a person can change the amount of acid that their stomach makes, alter the sensitivity of the gut and even modify the way the brain processes signals from the gut. In addition, it has the added benefit that it can be used to help in a psychological way by reducing stress and anxiety.

Many years ago we decided to see if hypnotherapy could be used to help with the management of IBS. We did a trial comparing what we call 'gut-focused hypnotherapy' with just talking to a person with IBS in a reassuring way, and found that those receiving the hypnotherapy improved much more than the other group. Since then we have done many more studies which have confirmed our original findings. Our results have also been reproduced by other researchers both in the UK and other countries. We find that overall approximately 70 per cent of people respond to treatment, with women responding a little better at 80 per cent and men not quite so well at 60 per cent. By response we mean a 50 per cent or more reduction in symptoms, so we never claim to cure IBS. It is very important that people accept that the tendency to develop gastrointestinal symptoms cannot be cured but that, with the aid of hypnotherapy, IBS can usually be brought under control.

One really interesting point about the response to hypnotherapy is that it improves all the symptoms of the condition, including the non-colonic symptoms (see page 36), which doesn't always happen with medication. It also reduces anxiety levels and if the sufferer has some depression that can also improve. There is no doubt that people thoroughly enjoy having a course of hypnotherapy treatment and usually don't want it to finish. However, it is most important that the person becomes independent of the therapist and learns how to use the technique on their own. To help with this they are given a CD with which to practise. It is essential that they practise regularly, especially at the beginning of treatment, as it is a skill you have to learn and, just like any other skill, the more you practise the better.

Treatment is best provided by an individual therapist at weekly intervals for a period of 6–12 weeks. If it hasn't helped after 12 weeks there is little point in continuing and it should be considered as unsuccessful. Fortunately, when hypnotherapy proves to be effective the benefits are nearly always permanent. However, some people require the occasional top-up which usually only involves one or two sessions. Some only require a top-up every few years whereas others may need one a little more frequently. In our Unit we do not allow regular top-ups as that encourages dependency and would also reduce the number of new IBS sufferers we could treat.

It would be nice if we could predict who is going to respond to treatment to save those destined to fail from disappointment. Unfortunately, we have never been able to find a reliable predictor of success and, therefore, we just have to try the treatment on everyone who wants to have it. However, there are absolutely no side-effects, so the worst that can happen is nothing and the best is a dramatic improvement in symptoms. Consequently, people have nothing to lose by trying this approach to treatment. We do not see hypnotherapy as a 'stand alone' treatment and feel strongly that it should be part of an integrated care package. This should involve education, diet, lifestyle advice and medication. When the treatment is particularly successful, medication can often be stopped altogether but it is perfectly acceptable if someone still wants to take their medication occasionally. For instance, they may want to take a laxative if constipated and, in diarrhoea-type IBS, they may want to still carry some loperamide with them, just to give them more confidence.

## What happens when you have hypnotherapy for your IBS?

In our Unit hypnotherapy is carried out on an individual basis by one of our therapists who are all trained to use what we call the 'gut-focused' technique.

The first session is a 'getting to know you' session, including a tutorial on IBS giving information on some of the abnormalities of gastrointestinal function that contribute to symptoms, such as hypersensitivity (see page 22) and excessive contraction of the gut muscles (see page 23). In addition, patients are given a description of the various techniques which can be used to correct these abnormalities and bring their IBS under control.

It is also useful to hear from someone with IBS how they visualise what is going on in their tummy, so that the therapist can help them to change this image in a positive way. For instance, if they have a lot of bloating they may imagine this to be like a balloon inflated inside their tummy. In this situation the balloon is called a 'metaphor' for bloating. Metaphors are frequently used by the hypnotherapist to help people control their symptoms. For instance, if someone has bloating and a hypnotherapist told them, under hypnosis, to make it go away, they would have some difficulty in knowing what to do. However, if the therapist said 'imagine your bloating to be caused by a balloon in your tummy' followed by 'you are now slowly deflating the balloon and your bloating is steadily getting better', the patient is more likely to get a response. This is because, by the use of a metaphor, the brain can activate the necessary systems to bring about change without the person actually knowing how to make this happen. Figure 8 shows some of the images that people have described to us with respect to their IBS – perhaps you may be able to relate to one of them?

Actual hypnosis starts at the second session. The person is hypnotised, usually by getting them to progressively relax their muscles in conjunction with calming their mind. This process can be helped by getting them to imagine a very relaxing scene, if they are able to visualise well. When they

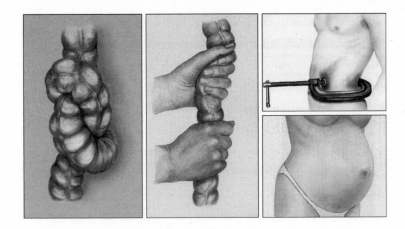

Figure 8 Many patients with IBS have a mental image of
their IBS – here are four examples

are sufficiently relaxed (in a trance) they can then start
learning how to bring their IBS under control by a variety
of techniques including metaphors.

For instance, they are asked to imagine their gut as a
river, the flow of which they are able to control by speeding
it up or slowing it down depending on what type of bowel
habit they have. In addition, they are asked to put their
hand on their tummy and feel a pleasant warming feeling
that can reach every part of their gut and give them control
over it. They are told that in the future every time they
put their hand on their tummy they will feel this warmth,
which will enable them to get rid of any pain. Eventually
they will be able to soothe their pain in day-to-day life by
just putting their hand on their tummy, without having to
go into a trance. At each session of treatment the process is
repeated and built upon according to the person's response.
The person does not speak during the session of hypnosis

and just listens to the therapist who does not ask any intrusive questions or require them to do anything unusual, other than to take control of their IBS – 'You will take control of your IBS, rather than it controlling you.' Each session takes approximately one hour and the process is repeated at weekly intervals, if possible, and is usually complete after 6–12 sessions. We always reassure our patients that we provide 'medical' hypnotherapy for their IBS and certainly do not want to explore their minds for hidden secrets or events. Our hypnotherapy is not a backward-looking form of treatment; we are only interested in moving forward.

CDs are provided with which to practice and this is an extremely important part of treatment. Daily practice is encouraged, which should be done at a time when patients won't immediately fall asleep. It is perfectly reasonable to use the CD to help with sleep, but it should also be used at another time to ensure that the full therapeutic effect is achieved.

As a person's symptoms improve they may be able to reduce their medication and even be a little more adventurous with their diet. However, they need to realise that their illness is under control and not cured, so there may still be some limitations on how far they can go.

# CHAPTER 9

# RECENT AND FUTURE DEVELOPMENTS

It is possible that some gastrointestinal conditions can give symptoms similar to IBS but be incorrectly diagnosed as IBS. This is important because, not only should we be making the right diagnosis, but also the alternative condition may be easier to treat than IBS. A good example of this is bile acid diarrhoea.

## Bile acid diarrhoea

Normally we make bile in the liver and it is passed into the bowel where it aids digestion by acting like a detergent (see page 5). Once the bile has done its job, it is reabsorbed by a part of the bowel called the terminal ileum (see page 9) and recirculated to the liver. However, the mechanism for reabsorbing bile can be faulty, or the liver can make too much bile so that it cannot all be reabsorbed. In both these situations the bile reaches the large bowel (colon) where it can cause diarrhoea (bile acid diarrhoea). Fortunately, there are medications that can bind to bile and stop it having an effect on the colon, which makes this condition very treatable. The two drugs that are used are called cholestyramine and colesevelam and it is well worth a person with the diarrhoea type of IBS trying one or other of these drugs. If you have bile acid diarrhoea, the response is very dramatic and the treatment should be continued at whatever dose best controls the symptoms. This can vary from person to person. Not surprisingly, some people have both bile acid diarrhoea and IBS, in which case the response might not be so good. In this situation it is only worth continuing with the bile acid treatment if it is making a worthwhile difference. Of course, some additional IBS treatment will probably be necessary under these circumstances. Some doctors recommend a test for bile acid diarrhoea called the SeHCAT test which is available in some hospitals. This is a perfectly reasonable suggestion but we prefer to just give the treatment, as the test is not always completely reliable.

## Small intestinal bacterial overgrowth (SIBO)

This is a rather controversial topic with some doctors strongly believing that it is a very important cause of IBS and others not being so convinced. Normally, the small bowel contains a relatively small number of bacteria but, if the motility (see page 11) of the gut becomes disordered, then the bacteria can build up to quite high levels. When this happens it can interfere with digestion and cause symptoms. This is called small intestinal bacterial overgrowth (SIBO) and can occur in diseases that can interfere with gastrointestinal function, such as diabetes or systemic sclerosis (a rare autoimmune disease) which affects the motility of the gut. It is also more likely to occur in people who either have low stomach acid or take medications that reduce acid such as the so-called proton pump inhibitors, for instance, omeprazole or lansoprazole.

With regard to SIBO and IBS, there are a number of problems in trying to work out what is going on. Firstly, the usual test for SIBO is a breath test following the consumption of a sugar, which is most often glucose. This test used to be done using lactulose but this is very unreliable and should not be used any more. Unfortunately, even when glucose is used, this is not a totally reliable test and can give a false positive result, but the glucose breath test is currently the best we have. Secondly, there is considerable variation in the number of bacteria in the small bowel even in people without IBS. So we don't exactly know when to call a result 'abnormal'. The third problem is that, even if SIBO is treated with an antibiotic, when the treatment is stopped the problem tends to reappear. This is presumably because the problem that is causing the SIBO is not put right by taking the antibiotic, which is just temporarily getting rid of the excess bacteria. Consequently, repeated courses of antibiotics will usually be needed and the long-term safety of such an approach has not yet been established. As the motility of the gut tends to be abnormal in IBS it seems reasonable to assume that SIBO is likely to occur, at least, in a proportion of sufferers.

If you do decide to try an antibiotic, then rifaximin is probably the best choice and you should take it for two weeks. This is an antibiotic that is not absorbed by the gut, which is a good thing because it just works on the gut bacteria. However, it is not available on an NHS prescription in the UK, although it can be obtained on a private prescription.

Some patients with IBS say that they have noticed that if they take an antibiotic for another reason, such as a chest infection, their IBS symptoms tend to improve. This observation suggests that bacteria are playing a part in that particular person's symptoms, but whether this is because they have SIBO or whether it has another explanation is unclear. People who experience this improvement often ask if they can have a repeat course of the antibiotic, but it does not always work a second time. If symptoms do improve, we then have the problem of whether it is safe to keep giving the antibiotic and that depends on balancing the risks of continuing the antibiotic compared to the severity of the IBS.

It is clear from the above that we still do not have all the answers about SIBO but, hopefully, future research will bring further clarification.

## Faecal transplantation

Despite some uncertainty about SIBO, there seems little doubt that, at least in some people with IBS, the bacteria in the gut, especially in the colon, are not entirely normal (see page 85). This is often referred to as dysbiosis. The exact cause of this is not known but it is probably relevant that a lot of IBS sufferers report that their symptoms seemed to start after an episode of gastroenteritis. In addition, a substantial number of people say that they have taken a lot of antibiotics in the past either as a child for problems like tonsillitis or as a teenager for acne. Consequently, these observations might at least partly explain why some people with IBS have dysbiosis.

One way to try and treat dysbiosis is with the use of probiotics and this has already been covered in Chapter 6. However, when the dysbiosis is very severe, it might be expecting too much for a single probiotic to have a meaningful effect as it is questionable whether the problem is just a deficiency of a single organism. It is much more likely that many bacteria might be deficient or abnormal. This raises the possibility that a better way of solving the problem would be to replace the whole microbiome and start afresh. One way of achieving this would be to transplant the faeces of a completely normal, healthy person into the bowel of someone with IBS, rather like we give a blood transfusion to someone who has lost blood.

There is a very dangerous condition called Clostridium difficile diarrhoea (C.diff diarrhoea) which can follow the use of antibiotics and in older people can be fatal. Faecal transplantation can nearly always cure this problem and this has resulted in people wondering whether it might be able to help a wide range of other gastrointestinal conditions, including IBS. The evidence that dysbiosis is a problem in IBS suggests that faecal transplantation might be worth trying in this condition and trials have already started. Obviously, transferring faeces from one person to another has potential dangers, such as the transfer of infection. Consequently, potential donors will have to be screened for transmittable diseases such as hepatitis, just as is currently undertaken in blood donors. In addition, we don't know whether one transplant is going to be sufficient or whether the process may need repeating and, if so, how many times. Lastly, donors are likely to vary in the composition of their microbiome, so it is possible that some donors may be more suitable for a particular disorder than others.

A faecal transplant is made from faeces which are lique-fied and then filtered. It can then be delivered either from below in the form of an enema or from above by running it down a tube which has been passed down the oesophagus though the stomach and into the small bowel. This avoids the stomach acid, which could kill some of the bacteria as well as the unpleasant possibility of it being regurgitated. It is probably better to give a transplant from above, as an enema is not going to reach very far into the bowel. However, many people are going to find the idea of a faecal transplant very unpleasant. This problem could be partly overcome by placing the material in capsules designed to not release their contents until they are well inside the small intestine and these are already being made available. In the very distant future it might be possible to create an artificial faecal transplant once we know which bacteria are the ones that need to be replaced in order to improve IBS. This would have the major advantage of being much more acceptable to patients as well as overcoming the potential problem of unwittingly transferring another disease to the recipient.

# CHAPTER 10

# IBS IN PREGNANCY, CHILDREN AND THE ELDERLY

Irritable bowel syndrome has no respect for age so it can affect the very young, the very old and all those in between.

## Pregnancy

There is some good news about pregnancy and IBS. Women with IBS are just as fertile as those without the condition and, in many, the symptoms improve during pregnancy and we certainly seldom see anyone getting worse. Consequently, IBS should not be seen as an obstacle to getting pregnant.

What concerns most women is whether it is safe to continue taking their medication while they are pregnant. Obviously, in an ideal world it is better to avoid any medication and, as IBS often improves in many people, this is frequently possible. However, in the more severe cases this is not always achievable and some realism has to creep in. Not surprisingly, and quite rightly, the medical profession are very nervous about the use of medication in pregnancy and you will never find a manufacturer of a medication who will say that their medication is safe during pregnancy.

Similarly, doctors frequently advise their IBS patients to stop their medication during pregnancy. However, we tell our patients that although we can't guarantee the safety of any particular medication there are some that, in our experience, do not seem to cause problems.

Antispasmodics such as mebeverine (Colofac) or hyoscine (Buscopan) appear to be safe but their use should be restricted to times when the pain is particularly severe. Severe diarrhoea needs to be brought under some degree of control and loperamide (Imodium) is the best choice. Some people use codeine to control both pain and diarrhoea but we advise against this as codeine is related to morphine and is addictive and can get into the baby's bloodstream.

Laxatives give us a particular problem as, in days gone by, large doses of laxatives have been used to try and induce an abortion. Consequently, there is the theoretical risk that laxatives might lead to a miscarriage. However, it is very important to not let women with IBS become very constipated during pregnancy because, eventually, they will need large doses of laxatives with an even greater risk of miscarriage. Our policy, in women who have anything more than mild constipation, is to encourage them to continue using their laxative throughout pregnancy. The preferred option for this purpose is macrogol (Movicol or Laxido).

Many women with the more severe forms of IBS are taking antidepressants, with the most common being amitriptyline. Many elect to come off this medication but in some this is impossible because of their symptom severity. There is little evidence that this particular antidepressant is harmful in pregnancy and, therefore, we give reassurance that they and their baby are extremely unlikely to come to any harm. There is less certainty about other antidepressants and in that situation, especially when they are being used for depression, we advise the women that they should discuss options with the doctor who is caring for this aspect of their health. The same goes for drugs that a woman might be taking for other conditions where there has to be a balance between the benefits and risks of continuing the medication during pregnancy.

## Children with IBS

Irritable bowel syndrome is very common in children and comes with its own challenges. When the child has the full range of symptoms the diagnosis is easy, but quite often they may have only one symptom, such as tummy pain or an unpredictable bowel habit, which leads to uncertainty. If investigation is negative and there is IBS in the family, that makes IBS more of a possibility. As a child gets older they tend to develop more typical symptoms which then makes the diagnosis more obvious.

Unfortunately, the symptoms can be just as severe as in adults and you can imagine how difficult it must be for a child to cope with pain which is as severe as labour pains in an adult female. Not surprisingly, schooling can be affected and the child might come under suspicion of faking the pain in order to avoid school. When the problem is diarrhoea the child may be reluctant to explain to staff the reason why they keep having to use the toilet. In addition, the reaction of teachers can be extremely important, as many may not be aware of just how bad the symptoms of IBS can be. Consequently, it is vital that there is good communication between parent and teacher and, if necessary, the doctor needs to become involved in this process. Irritable bowel syndrome should not cause failure to thrive in children and does not affect the onset of puberty. However, puberty can lead to a change in symptoms such as the bowel habit changing from loose to constipated.

The reaction of parents when a child is in pain is also very important, as they usually feel completely helpless when they see their child rolling about in pain. Therefore, they need to fully understand the situation and, once the diagnosis is secure, resist the temptation to keep taking their child to the A&E department, especially as they may be subjected to more unnecessary tests and even something like the unnecessary removal of their appendix if the pain is on the right side. Interestingly, it has been shown that if parents are too overprotective of children with IBS the children don't do as well as those who are dealt with in a more firm but sympathetic way.

Fortunately, the outlook is very good in most children with IBS and they can usually be managed with the same medications that are used in adults. Sometimes antidepressants have to be used which usually meets with considerable hesitancy from the parents. Consequently, it is important to emphasise that the medication is being used at a low dose to target the gut rather than the head. Parents are also often keen to give their offspring as healthy a diet as possible and this may not be such a good idea in IBS where perhaps some moderation is best advised, usually to the child's delight. The sooner the IBS can be brought under control the better, as there is evidence that the longer a person has uncontrolled symptoms the more difficult it is to bring IBS under control in the future.

In a child with IBS who does not respond to the usual measures, hypnotherapy can be a particularly good treatment option with an extremely high success rate because children have an especially good imagination.

## IBS in the elderly

As we get older we are more likely to develop a whole range of diseases and doctors are well aware that an older person with symptoms is more likely to be suffering from something serious like cancer. Consequently if, for instance, an older person complains of abdominal pain, constipation, bloating, low backache, constant lethargy, nausea and bladder symptoms (the typical picture of IBS), the doctor is going to worry that something sinister is going on. In this situation it is absolutely essential to do all the necessary tests to exclude anything serious but if they all turn out to be negative then the diagnosis of IBS has to be seriously considered. This can then prevent a merry-go-round of unnecessary repetitive investigation and stress for all concerned. Unfortunately, this does not always happen in the elderly.

Once a diagnosis is established, the treatment is exactly the same as for younger IBS sufferers and can be very welcome in someone who has often been subjected to a whole variety of investigation but offered little in the way of treatment.

# CHAPTER 11

# QUESTIONS AND ANSWERS

**Q.** I have been told I have got a spastic bowel. Is this the same as IBS?

**A.** Yes, over the years IBS has been given a lot of different names and these are listed in Table 14. However, these other names are now being used less and less and we should be sticking to the name irritable bowel syndrome.

---

**Table 14** Names that have been used for IBS

- Spastic colon bowel
- Mucous colitis
- Irritable colon
- Colospasm
- Spastic constipation
- Painless diarrhoea
- Enterospasm
- Enteralgia
- Membranous colitis
- Abdominal migraine

---

**Q.** Can my IBS be cured?

**A.** No, but in the vast majority of people it can be brought under control so that it becomes a bit of a nuisance rather than a constant intrusion.

**Q.** Can IBS lead to cancer?

**A.** No.

**Q.** Will my IBS get worse as I get older?

**A.** No, it is unlikely to get worse and usually improves. Irritable bowel syndrome seems to be particularly troublesome between the age of 15 and 30.

**Q.** Does exercise help IBS?

**A.** Yes, but it should not be too vigorous. Strenuous exercise can sometimes make IBS more troublesome particularly if you have the diarrhoea version.

**Q.** Do men get IBS?

**A.** Yes, but their symptoms can differ from those of women. The bowel habit in men is more often loose than consti-pated and they do not seem to bloat quite as much as women.

**Q.** What is indigestion?

**A.** Doctors are trying not to use this term anymore as it is so vague and means different things to different people. For instance, one person might call their tummy pain indigestion where others may use the term to describe heartburn or nausea.

**Q.** My stools float and are difficult to flush away. Is this abnormal?

**A.** No, it is because they contain some trapped air. You should only be concerned about floating stools if they are loose, very greasy and very pale in colour (like clay). When they are like this it can be a sign that you are not absorbing food properly.

**Q.** My stools sometimes contain undigested food like peas or nuts. Is this a problem?

**A.** No, finding bits of food in your stools, especially if your bowels tend to be rather loose, is very unlikely to indicate a problem. Sweetcorn is commonly visible in stools and can even be used as a rough measure of how quickly food is going through you, although it can sometimes upset people with IBS.

**Q.** Can some foods look like blood in my stools?

**A.** Yes, this is quite a common cause of people thinking they have blood in their stools. Tomatoes, red peppers, beetroot and raspberries are particular offenders. However, it is vital that blood in the stool is not ignored, so if there is any doubt, consult your doctor.

**Q.** Why does my bottom itch so much, particularly at night?

**A.** Many patients with IBS have an itchy bottom (pruritus ani). It is more common in people with a loose bowel habit as this can lead to some inflammation of the skin around the anus. The itching can be worse at night and some people even wake up to find themselves scratching their bottom which makes it even more sore and itchy. The treatment is to preferably wash your bottom with soap and water after each bowel opening and possibly use a soothing cream from the chemist. Occasionally, a mild steroid-containing cream may be necessary. Threadworms can cause an itchy bottom, especially in children, but this is much less likely to be the cause of the problem in adults.

**Q.** How long is it safe to go without opening my bowels?

**A.** We see lots of people who don't open their bowels for two weeks or more. However, it is not a good idea to leave your bowels unopened for this long although it is extremely unlikely to do you any harm. Consequently, in such a situation we always recommend that you should take a regular laxative with the aim of trying to keep your bowels open as often as possible. We aim for every day but this is not always achievable.

**Q.** Is it safe to take a laxative all the time?

**A.** Yes, there is no evidence to suggest that laxatives such as macrogol (Movicol, Laxido) damage the bowel or make it lazier than it is already. The best way to take a laxative is to take the lowest dose that works for you, on a daily basis, to try and mimic a normal bowel habit as far as possible. Taking a laxative regularly results in a much more predictable bowel habit than taking it intermittently. If you only take a laxative intermittently, you often need a bigger dose which can then result in a more unpredictable and sometimes rather explosive result.

**Q.** Which is best, laxatives or suppositories?

**A.** Whichever suits you best. Laxatives are usually needed for the more stubborn forms of constipation and there is nothing to stop you using them both together.

**Q.** Can massage help constipation?

**A.** Yes, some people find that massaging the colon (see Figure 1 on page 7) in the direction of flow of its contents from right to left, can be helpful.

**Q.** Can smoking help constipation?

**A.** Yes, but it should not be advised because of all the health problems associated with smoking. An appropriate dose of a laxative is a far better and safer option.

**Q.** If my general practitioner gives me an antibiotic for a particular problem, my IBS seems to improve. Why is this?

**A.** It is not uncommon for people with IBS to notice this and it probably indicates that the bacteria in your gut are not quite normal which is known to happen in some patients with IBS. If this happens, it is tempting to try antibiotics for the IBS (see page 117) but the safety of taking them long term is not known.

**Q.** Is it worth trying probiotics for my IBS?

**A.** Yes, they can be helpful (see page 85). Probiotics are harmless bacteria which seem to improve the symptoms of IBS in some patients. They don't work instantly and are probably best for the milder forms of IBS. They are very safe and may have other benefits such as improving the function of your immune system. They are most commonly available in yoghurts and milk-based drinks but are also obtainable in capsule form, which is helpful for those people who have problems with milk products. The commonest organisms used are various varieties of bifidobacteria and lactobacilliae with bifidobacteria appearing to be somewhat more effective in IBS.

**Q.** We are told that bowel (colon) cancer is quite common and that the first symptom is often a change of bowel habit and rectal bleeding. I have IBS and am 60 years old with an unpredictable bowel habit and some bleeding when I am constipated. How would I know if I have developed bowel cancer?

**A.** This is a concern. Hopefully, there will soon be a stool test that will help to detect bowel cancer. Until that time you should be alert to any change in your usual symptom pattern and any bleeding that is not associated with any anal symptoms. Darker coloured blood should always be taken more seriously. If you have a family history of bowel cancer, that should be reported to your doctor. After the age of 60, there is a national screening programme for bowel cancer in the UK which tests the stool for microscopic amounts of blood (faecal occult blood test) which can happen with bowel cancer. However, if you have visible rectal bleeding this will give you a positive result as the test is designed to detect any amount of blood. Consequently, the result will be more reliable if you do the test when you are not bleeding at all and you don't even have a sore bottom, because that can also lead to a small amount of blood in the stools. If you are concerned about this problem, you should consult your doctor about having a colonoscopy which is the best test for detecting bowel cancer. It is very important to detect bowel cancer at the early stage as this form of cancer has a particularly good outlook if treated early.

**Q.** What is an endoscopy?

**A.** An endoscopy is a general term for any procedure where a camera on a telescope is passed into the body. In the field of gastroenterology, a gastroscopy is when the telescope is passed through your mouth into your stomach and duodenum (see Figure 1 on page 7) and a colonoscopy is when the telescope is passed through your anus and around your colon. These two tests are nearly always done under sedation rather than a general anaesthetic. Some brave people choose to have the test without any sedation. Gynaecologists often perform a laparoscopy in order to inspect the outside of the womb and ovaries. In this procedure, which is done under general anaesthetic, the telescope is passed through a small cut made in the tummy button (umbilicus). Laparoscopy is sometimes requested by gastroenterologists, especially when they are suspicious there may be a gynaecological cause for the patient's symptoms. More recently, a camera in the form of a disposable capsule can be swallowed to allow inspection of the small bowel (capsule endoscopy).

**Q.** What is a gastroenterologist?

**A.** This is a physician (not a surgeon) who specialises in gastrointestinal problems. These days a gastroenterologist who specialises in liver problems is usually called a hepatologist. A surgeon who specialises in gastrointestinal problems is usually called a gastrointestinal surgeon and these often divide themselves into 'upper' and 'lower' gastrointestinal surgeons. A lower gastrointestinal surgeon is sometimes called a colorectal surgeon.

**Q.** I have IBS and there is IBS in my family. Is there anything I can do to minimise the chances of my children getting IBS?

**A.** Irritable bowel syndrome does run in families but that does not mean that every child will develop the problem. If one of your children starts complaining of suggestive symptoms then it would be a good idea to get the diagnosis confirmed. Once confirmed, then treatment as outlined in the various chapters of this book should be started, as the sooner a child learns how to control the problem the better. Hypnotherapy is particularly good for children with IBS.

**Q.** I sometimes can't seem to be able to get enough air into my lungs. What is the problem?

**A.** This is a symptom of hyperventilation (over-breathing). Hyperventilation is quite common in people with IBS and can make their symptoms worse. Relaxation and breathing exercises can help this problem.

**Q.** What is the difference between an allergy and an intolerance?

**A.** An allergy is an immunological reaction to something to which you have particular antibodies (IgE antibodies). The commonest example is hay fever. Food allergies are more common in people with eczema, asthma and hay fever and there is a very rapid reaction (sometimes within minutes) when the offending food is swallowed. This can include abdominal pain, itching, urticaria (hives), swelling of the lips, tongue or face and even breathlessness, which can be severe. A food intolerance is not due to an immunological reaction and comes on much more slowly than an allergy. It is thought that reactions to food in people with IBS are mainly due to food intolerances rather than allergies despite the fact that hay fever, eczema and asthma are more common in IBS.

**Q.** Can herbal remedies or Traditional Chinese Medicine help IBS?

**A.** There is some emerging evidence that these approaches may be helpful in IBS but experience of their use within the NHS is very limited and more research is needed before a definite answer to this question can be given.

**Q.** Can acupuncture help IBS?

**A.** The evidence that acupuncture helps IBS is rather conflicting but some people, especially those with the milder forms of IBS, seem to derive some benefit from it. Therefore, as long as a safe and competent practitioner delivers the acupuncture, it may be worth trying especially if you are making no progress with conventional approaches.

**Q.** I get a lot of bad breath. Could this be related to my IBS?

**A.** There is no doubt that many patients with IBS say they have bad breath, especially if they have the constipation variety of IBS. Obviously poor dental hygiene can lead to bad breath but most people with IBS actually take good care of their teeth, so it is unlikely that the problem is coming from dental or gum disease. Bad breath can result from a lack of saliva, which normally keeps the mouth flushed out and also has the capacity to kill smell-producing bacteria with the enzymes it contains. Some people with IBS tend to have a dry mouth so lack of saliva may be contributing to bad breath in these individuals. In addition, some of the medications used in IBS can also cause a dry mouth. It is also known that some of the gases produced in the gut, which may smell, can get into the bloodstream and reach the lungs where they pass into the breath. This is another possible explanation for some cases of bad breath. However, until we actually know what causes this problem in IBS, it is difficult to recommend a solution. Consequently, it is our policy to concentrate on treating the IBS and we usually find that if the IBS improves, then the bad breath also often improves. Some people try chewing gum to stop bad breath but we usually advise against this for several reasons. Firstly, because even chewing on its own can make IBS worse, secondly, because the resulting increased swallowing can lead to accumulation of gas and, lastly, because the artificial sweeteners in the chewing gum can also cause excess gas production (see page 16).

**Q.** Does IBS cause an unpleasant taste in the mouth?

**A.** Yes, it can do and some people say it tastes rather metallic.

**Q.** I am a diabetic and the advice the diabetic team are giving me conflicts with what the gastroenterologist is telling me.

**A.** There is no doubt that some of the foods that are considered healthy tend to upset the tummy of some people with IBS. However, it is very important that people with diabetes do adhere to a healthy diet as, in contrast to IBS, diabetes is associated with long-term complications. Consequently, we usually advise people with IBS and diabetes to try cutting back on some, but not necessarily all, of the healthy foods and reaching a compromise. In other words, we do not advise them to eat unhealthily, but alert them to the fact that some of the more healthy foods may upset their tummy. There is nothing worse than being given conflicting advice from two different medical teams. Consequently, if possible, it is a good idea to try and get the two teams liaising over your care, although this is not always possible.

**Q.** I am a vegetarian and am not prepared to change my diet, even if it might help my IBS.

**A.** Although manipulating the diet can be useful in many patients with IBS it does not, by any means, help everyone. Even when dietary measures do prove helpful the response is seldom complete and this is because a whole variety of factors can influence the severity of the condition. Therefore, if someone would rather not change their diet they can always try other approaches such as medication or behavioural treatment.

**Q.** Why does my bottom get so sore?

**A.** This is very common in people with a loose bowel habit due to the loose stool inflaming the skin. If possible, it is preferable to wash your bottom after every bowel movement. In addition, a barrier cream applied to a clean bottom is helpful, particularly if you are unable to wash after every bowel movement. In people with constipation and hard stools, the stool can be hard enough to split the skin of the anus which then becomes sore. This is called an anal fissure and the typical symptom is a sharp pain in the anus during the passage of a hard stool, followed by some bleeding. If there is bleeding without pain or soreness of your bottom you should consult your doctor.

**Q.** I sometimes feel a pulsation or a vibrating sensation in my bowel. Is this normal?

**A.** Some people with IBS mention these sensations and they are nothing to worry about and are part of having an oversensitive tummy (see hypersensitivity, page 22). Some older people worry that the pulsation could mean they have an aortic aneurysm but this is extremely unlikely. However, if you are concerned about this, it is best to get your doctor to examine your tummy to check this out. The aorta is a large artery running down through the body from the heart to the pelvis. An aortic aneurysm is a swelling of the aorta which happens when the artery wall becomes weakened.

**Q.** I have been told that I have IBS but I do not get any bloating. Does this mean I could have something different?

**A.** Although the majority of people with IBS get bloating, some people do not experience this symptom. Similarly, some people with IBS have a normal bowel habit but lots of bloating and pain or no pain but an abnormal bowel habit and bloating. When a patient has all the symptoms of pain, bloating and an abnormal bowel habit, the diagnosis is easy. When someone has only two symptoms, the doctor has to be more careful and do more tests. However, if the tests rule out anything else, then it is reasonable to conclude the symptoms are due to IBS. Diagnosis becomes much more difficult in someone who only has one symptom, but we do see patients who just get pain. If the pain is twisting or squeezing which is typical of IBS and there is no evidence of any other gastrointestinal disorder, it is reasonable to treat it as a case of gastrointestinal spasm.

It is now being recognised that there are many people in the general population who experience 'minor digestive symptoms' which are not sufficient to make a diagnosis of IBS. It seems reasonable to assume that the gastrointestinal system can give symptoms now and again without necessarily meaning that there is anything wrong with it, just like if a person gets a headache it doesn't mean they have got migraine. However, it could be that at least some of these people might have very mild cases of IBS, who might get more symptoms if they were unfortunate enough to encounter a trigger that could make them worse (see page 21).

**Q.** I had an episode of gastroenteritis about a month ago and am still getting some symptoms. Could it be IBS?

**A.** Gastroenteritis is a well-recognised trigger for IBS, but not all people who get gastroenteritis or food poisoning develop IBS. It is surprising how long it can take to recover completely from such an event. We do not even start to suspect IBS for at least three months and frequently see people who can take up to six months for their symptoms to completely disappear after a gastrointestinal infection. The same rules apply to diarrhoea which has been brought on by antibiotics.

**Q.** What is campylobacter?

**A.** Campylobacter is a type of bacteria, which is the commonest cause of gastroenteritis in the UK. Symptoms include abdominal pain, diarrhoea which can be blood-stained, a temperature and sometimes vomiting. Other bacteria that commonly cause gastroenteritis in the UK are salmonella and shigella. When bacterial gastroenteritis is severe it is sometimes called dysentery and in other countries dysentery can be caused by other organisms such as amoebae (amoebic dysentery). Viruses can also cause gastroenteritis with norovirus (winter vomiting virus) being the most common in adults and rotavirus the most common in children. Gastroenteritis is important in relation to IBS because it can make IBS worse or possibly even trigger it off in the first place. When IBS is triggered by gastroenteritis it is sometimes called 'post-infective IBS' or 'post-dysenteric IBS'.

**Q.** I have been told I have got H. pylori infection. Is this causing my IBS?

**A.** There is no evidence that H. pylori causes IBS. It is a germ that only inhabits the stomach and can lead to an ulcer but not IBS. It has been suggested that it may cause upper gastrointestinal symptoms but not everyone agrees with this opinion. It can usually be eradicated by a cocktail of strong antibiotics, but the ones used can sometimes lead to a temporary deterioration in IBS.

**Q.** What is the difference between an acute and chronic medical condition?

**A.** The words 'acute' and 'chronic' are often used differently by the medical profession and the public. Patients often use the word chronic to imply severity of a symptom or condition, whereas to a doctor chronic just means it is a long-standing condition and has no meaning with regard to severity. An acute condition or symptom has a sudden onset and only lasts a short or relatively short period of time. Consequently, IBS is a chronic condition.

**Q.** My IBS gives me so many different symptoms I don't know what to tell my doctor in a ten-minute appointment.

**A.** This can be a problem. It is best to tell them your worst symptoms even if they are embarrassing. Many patients don't mention their faecal incontinence which is a mistake as this is probably the one that will convince the doctor the most that you need help. Rather than just saying the pain is severe, if you are female and have had a baby, you could say it is similar to labour pains, or worse! Doctors tend to not take bloating very seriously, so if you are someone who looks pregnant by the evening, take a photograph of it to show them. The non-colonic symptoms of IBS (see page 58) can be very intrusive but many doctors who are not specialists in IBS are not aware of how much of a problem they can be. Constant tiredness and lethargy can be a major problem in IBS, but, many doctors are more aware of lethargy being a symptom of depression than IBS, so they may decide that you are depressed if you mention this symptom. Depression is uncommon in IBS and it is important that you realise that the lethargy of IBS is far more likely to be due to the IBS than depression.

**Q.** What is the difference between a CT scan and an MRI scan?

**A.** They are both very sophisticated ways of picturing the internal organs of the body. The main difference is that a CT (Computerised Tomography) scan uses X-rays and an MRI (Magnetic Resonance Imaging) scan uses a magnet.

**Q.** My IBS is so bad that I can't work any more. Am I entitled to any benefits?

**A.** Disability benefits are usually offered to people who can't walk, climb stairs or who suffer from symptoms such as severe breathlessness. Consequently, the benefits system does not really have a reliable mechanism for determining disability related to gastrointestinal disorders and, therefore, many people with severe IBS have great difficulty in accessing disability benefits.

**Q.** Is IBS any more common in people with learning difficulties?

**A.** Probably not, but that still means that as many as 15 per cent of such people will have IBS by chance because about 15 per cent of the population have IBS and people with learning difficulties are no exception to this rule. Irritable bowel syndrome can be very difficult to manage in this situation especially when communication is limited. If someone with learning difficulties is regularly looking distressed and holding their tummy, it is well worth considering the diagnosis of IBS.

# CONCLUSION

If not brought under control, IBS can become a miserable condition with which to live and can affect every aspect of a sufferer's life. In addition to the typical, well-known, features of abdominal pain, an abnormal bowel habit and bloating, people with IBS often suffer from one or more non-colonic symptoms which can make the condition even more intrusive. These include constant lethargy, low backache, nausea, bladder symptoms, chest pain, thigh pain and joint or muscle pains. Women with IBS have the added burden of suffering pain on intercourse as well as their tummy pain often being made worse by their periods. Not surprisingly, general practitioners are often baffled by someone complaining of such a wide range of symptoms and, if one of the non-colonic symptoms is particularly prominent, may send them to the wrong specialty. Consequently, sufferers can, for instance, end up in a gynaecological clinic where there is the possibility that they may have unnecessary investigations or even surgery. Other clinics to which people with IBS can be wrongly referred include orthopaedics (backache), rheumatology (joint pains), urology (bladder symptoms), cardiology (chest pain), haematology (lethargy) and endocrinology (lethargy). Unfortunately, if the sufferer's journey through the healthcare system starts in the wrong clinic, they may be subjected to a whole variety of tests and treatments which may be unnecessary and can even make their symptoms worse. Women with IBS often say that the pain can be worse than that of childbirth, therefore, it is not surprising that with pain of that intensity sufferers have to go to A&E departments where, again, the real cause of their pain may not be recognised and they are just given morphine. All this highlights the vital importance of the correct diagnosis being made as early as possible, so that the appropriate treatment is started as soon as possible.

Contrary to popular belief, IBS can be managed effectively in the vast majority of cases but what helps one person may not help another, even if they have similar symptoms. Consequently, one size does not fit all and inevitably treatment has to be a process of trial and error until a treatment plan that suits the particular individual is found. Similarly, a combination of treatments is often required to achieve the optimum benefit. However, it is important to introduce one treatment at a time otherwise it is impossible to determine what has worked and what has not.

Diet is extremely important and it is rather unusual for someone to not make any progress at all with dietary manipulation. Unfortunately, a very healthy diet can actually make IBS worse and sufferers often find this a difficult concept to accept, especially with all the encouragement we are given to eat healthily. For someone with a normal gut, healthy eating is absolutely fine and should be encouraged, but unfortunately the oversensitive gut of IBS tends to groan if given too much cereal fibre, fruit or vegetables. That doesn't mean to say that we are advocating unhealthy eating, it is just that it is important to be aware that some so-called healthy foods may upset a particular person. Therefore, each person needs to work out which are their 'safe' and 'unsafe' foods, so that when they are going through a bad phase they can limit themselves to their safer foods until things settle down again.

With regard to abdominal pain, antispasmodics are the first line of treatment and it is often best to try a variety to find out which one suits you best. Laxatives do not damage the bowel and the best way to take them is regularly at the lowest dose that controls the problem. Similarly, loperamide (Imodium) is very safe for diarrhoea although some people say that it can sometimes make discomfort or bloating a little worse. It is acceptable to take loperamide on an 'as necessary' or regular basis or even before an event that you think might cause you trouble with your bowels.

When IBS cannot be controlled by diet, antispasmodics, laxatives or antidiarrhoeals, it is perfectly reasonable to try an antidepressant as these medications can also have an effect on the gut. For IBS, the most commonly used antidepressant is a low-dose tricyclic antidepressant such as amitriptyline. The main side-effects are dry mouth, sleepiness and sometimes constipation. These usually wear off after a week or two but it is best to always take the medication at night to help deal with any sleepiness. In fact, the sleepiness can be an advantage in people who do not sleep very well. If someone is constipated, they can still take this medication but may have to increase the dose of their laxative. If somebody can't tolerate a tricyclic antidepressant, then an SSRI (see page 88) is worth considering, especially if the constipation continues to be a problem, as this group of antidepressants can actually lead to a slightly loose bowel habit. At the doses we use, the tricyclic antidepressants do not have much antidepressant activity and if someone is particularly depressed then an SSRI is a better choice. If we are not sure, we sometimes ask the patient whether they want us to target their head or their gut. In many people the depression is a result of their IBS and then it is best to target the gut.

If these measures don't help, then behavioural approaches such as hypnotherapy, CBT or psychotherapy should be considered and are frequently very effective.

Even when all the measures that are described above are not effective, there are other approaches that can be used to improve the problem, but these are only available in specialised centres such as ours and are really beyond the scope of this book, which is aimed at encouraging self-help.

There is now a lot of research going on into IBS and, as we learn more about the condition, it is inevitable that better ways of managing it will emerge. However, even today with all the approaches that have been described in this book, the majority of sufferers can be put 'back on track' and it is hoped that this short book will help you to take control of your IBS.

Good luck!

# INDEX